A Group of Experienced Family Medicine and Internal Medicine Consultants

Adil Alharti, Khalid Almutairi

Pitfalls in Family Medicine Clinical Practice

AUSTIN MACAULEY PUBLISHERS™
LONDON * CAMBRIDGE * NEW YORK * SHARJAH

Copyright © Adil Alharti, Khalid Almutairi 2024

The right of Adil Alharti, Khalid Almutairi to be identified as author of this work has been asserted by the author in accordance with Federal Law No. (7) of UAE, Year 2002, Concerning Copyrights and Neighboring Rights.

All rights reserved. No part of this publication may be reproduced, stored in a retrieval system, or transmitted in any form or by any means, electronic, mechanical, photocopying, recording, or otherwise, without the prior permission of the publishers.

Any person who commits any unauthorized act in relation to this publication may be liable to legal prosecution and civil claims for damages.

The age group that matches the content of the books has been classified according to the age classification system issued by the Ministry of Culture and Youth.

ISBN 9789948762133 (Paperback)
ISBN 9789948762140 (E-Book)

Application Number: MC-10-01-2852480
Age Classification: E

Printer Name: iPrint Global Ltd
Printer Address: Witchford, England

First Published 2024
AUSTIN MACAULEY PUBLISHERS FZE
Sharjah Publishing City
P.O Box [519201]
Sharjah, UAE
www.austinmacauley.ae
+971 655 95 202

Sara A. Alharthi, medical student of Ibn Sina National College of Medical Studies for her active role in pre-submission proofreading.

Table of Contents

Preface	9
Fever Chapter	10
Back Pain Chapter	40
Neurological Presentations	77
Arthralgia Chapter	89
Dementia Chapter	113
Blue Mood Chapter	130
Lower Limb Edema Chapter	142
Palpitation Chapter	158
Urinary Incontinence	172
Dyspnea Chapter	191

Preface

Over the last few years, the discipline of general practice has been developed greatly. A general practitioner needs a broad base of knowledge and a wide range of skills to take care of his patients.

Within a busy time, limited consultation, the general practitioner must do his best to approach different patient complaints and decide the appropriate management plan.

Consultation is the heart of general practice. We have constructed a clinical case-scenario based on the real-life practice of a group of family medicine and internal medicine senior physicians.

Our cases are designed to be symptom-based where we tackle the common and important presenting symptoms in our practice.

The case scenarios are designed to be a dialogue between the physician and his patients, we tried to pick up mistakes which may happen during the consultation and then correct the approach to be ideal, the mistakes are listed and a take home message was elaborated at the end of each case.

We are looking for your kind feedback for any ideas for improvement, wishing to you a successful practice.

Fever Chapter

MOHAMMED M. AL ASMARI, MD
SARA M. ABOLLEIF, MD

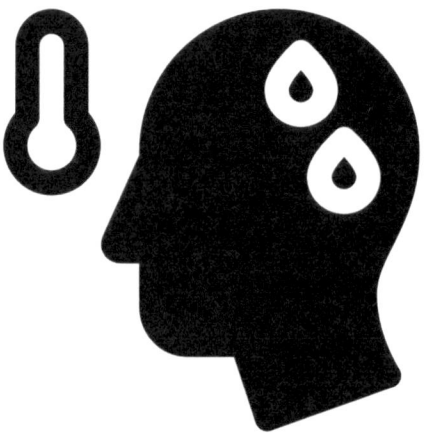

Case Study 1

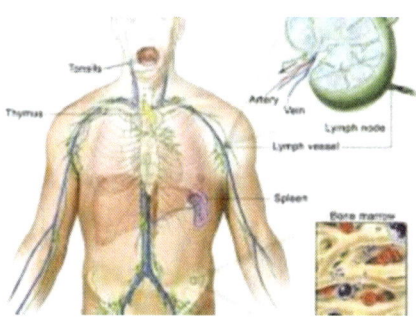

A 16-year-old male patient student in intermediate school presented with his father to the Family Medicine Clinic complaining of fever.

Physician: When did the fever start?
Father: According to his mother approximately one to two weeks but I am not sure.

Physician: Any contact with Covid patients?
Father: No.

Physician saw patient's throat by inspection and no redness was seen.
Physician: Okay I think your son has only URTI, he needs amoxicillin, paracetamol and bed rest.

What went wrong in the previous scenario?
- Physician did not introduce himself.
- Physician did not ask the patient about his name to establish good rapport with him.
- Physician took history from father which is not right, he should take it from the patient.

- Did not take the permission to examine the patient.
- Did not take detailed history of fever (degree of fever, nature of fever, response to antipyretics, associated symptoms including weight loss and lose appetite and night sweats…).
- Did not do proper clinical examination including GPE* and focused clinical examination.

Ideal Scenario

A 16-year-old male patient, student in intermediate school presented with his father to Family Medicine Clinic complaining of fever.

Physician: Salaam Alaikum, I am Doctor Tariq. What is your name?
Patient: Khalid.

Physician: How are you Khalid?
Father: He complains of fever.

Physician: I asked Khalid.
Father: Okay.
Patient: I have a fever.
Physician: Since when?
Patient: Three weeks to one month.

Physician: Is it intermittent or continuous?
Patient: It is continuous especially at night.

Physician: Is it responding to antipyretics?
Patient: No.

Physician: Is there a night sweat?
Patient: Yes.

Physician: Do you have weight loss?
Patient: Yes, I lost 15 kg in the last 6 months.

Physician: Have you lost appetite?
Patient: Yes.

Physician: Did you notice any swelling or lumps in the body?
Patient: I noticed swelling in Right axilla.

Physician: When did you notice this swelling?
Patient: I think three to four months.

Physician: Are there other swellings?
Patient: No.

Physician: Do you smoke?
Patient: Yes, half packet daily.

Physician: Did you travel recently?
Patient: No.

Physician: Do you have animal exposure?
Patient: No.

Physician: Okay, Khaild, so your complaint in summary:
You are a 16-year-old male student in secondary school complaining of fever for the last 3-4 weeks continuously not responding to antipyretics associated with weight loss and loss of appetite and night sweats and you noticed swelling in your right axilla.

Physician: Do you want to add other information?
Patient: No.
Father: Yes doctor, his uncle had cancer two years ago.

Physician: What type of cancer?
Father: We don't know.

Physician: What is your concern, Khalid?
Father: We want to know what is his problem.

Physician: I asked Khalid.
Patient: I want something to relieve the fever.

Physician: What do you expect from me?
Patient: I want to know why the fever is not resolving.

Physician: Okay! Khalid, I want to examine you. Do you allow me?
Patient: Yes.

During the Examination:

Temperature: 38.3, pulse: 99b/min regular, BP: 108/70, O2 sat: 99% RA*, weight: 61 kg, Height: 155 cm.

Lymph Node Exam:

- Cervical LN: there is palpable LN in right cervical area about 1X1.5 cm, hard, nontender, fixed.
- Axillary LN: there is palpable LN in the right axilla about 2X2 cm, hard, nontender, fixed.
- Supraclavicular, epitrochlear, inguinal popliteal LN: NO PALPABLE LN.

Discussion and Counseling:

Physician: Okay Khalid, after taking history and physical exam, I think we need more investigation to know what is the reason for this fever?
Patient: What can you offer me doctor?

Physician: Okay, I will request Basic labs...CBC, Coagulation profile, Biochemistry labs, Uric acid, LDH, CRP, ESR. You also need U/S (Ultra sound) of the right axilla.
Physician: Regarding fever, I will prescribe for you paracetamol 1 gm, every 8 hours PRN* to settle the fever.

Patient: Okay, doctor.

Labs Results:

CBC showed mild normocytic normochromic anemia.

Biochemistry showed high LDH and ESR.

U/S Axilla showed 2x2 cm echogenic LN.

Physician explained the results of investigation to the patient and his father and the need to do LN biopsy for diagnosis.

Physician refers him to General surgeon for Biopsy to be done.

Biopsy came as Hodgkin lymphoma.

Physician: Okay, Khalid let me explain to you what we have to do now.
Patient: Okay, doctor.

Physician starts to break bad news.

Physician closes clinic room to achieve privacy for the patient. Physician closes his mobile to minimize interruption and calls nurse staff to attend the discussion and for documentation.

Physician: Do you want anybody with you?
Patient: Yes, my father.

Physician: Okay, Khalid.
Father came.

Physician: Okay, Khalid, what do you know so far?
Patient: Nothing, I did labs and LN biopsy.

Physician: Do you know why we have been doing these tests?
Patient: Yes, you want to know the reason of the fever.
Physician: Good

Physician: Are you the sort of person who likes to know all the available facts?
Father: Yes, doctor.
Patient: Yes.

Physician: I am afraid the test results show that things are more serious than we thought.

Father: What do you mean by serious?

Physician: Some cells look abnormal.
Father: Do you mean he has cancer?

Physician: Yes.
Physician allows the information to sink in and he gives time to show emotions
Father: What can we do now, Doctor?

Physician: Okay, I will help you as much as I can. I will refer you to the oncology department in our hospital, and he will explain to you what the plan of management is.
Father: Okay! Thank you, Doctor!
Physicians now summarize the information given, check their understanding, repeat any information as necessary, allow time for questions, and then make arrangements with the oncology physician to see the patient on an urgent basis.

Physician: Do you understand everything that I have discussed?
Patient and Father: Yes.

Physician: Is there anything that you would like to ask?
Father: Yes, when should we see an oncology physician?

Physician: Yes, I made arrangements with him. He will see you tomorrow morning in the oncology clinic.
Physician: Do you want to ask any other questions?
Father and Patient: No! Thanks, Dr. Tariq.

Differential Diagnosis of Lymphadenopathy:

Localized or regional lymphadenopathy	Infections (involving skin, oral maxillary and genitourinary, e.g. lymphogranuloma venereum caused by *Chlamydia trachomatis*)
	'Cat scratch disease' infection with the bacterium *Bartonella henselae* causes painful enlarged regional lymphadenopathy associated with fever
	Primary haematological malignancy, e.g. Hodgkin's lymphoma, which typically spreads contiguously, i.e. 'from one lymph node to another'
	Other malignancies metastasizing to lymph nodes by local or distant spread
Generalized lymphadenopathy	Infections, e.g. viral (Epstein–Barr virus, cytomegalovirus, human immunodeficiency virus, rubella), bacterial (tuberculosis, syphilis) or protozoal (toxoplasmosis, leishmaniasis)
	Lymphoproliferative and myeloproliferative disorders
	Autoimmune (e.g. systemic lupus erythematosus, rheumatoid arthritis, Sjögren's syndrome)
	Dermatopathic (e.g. eczema, psoriasis)
	Drugs (e.g. allopurinol, carbamazepine, phenytoin, penicillins, atenolol, captopril, isoniazid)

Table 1: Causes of Lymphadenopathy

Clinical Pearls and Take-Home Messages

- Lymphoma classified into Non-Hodgkin lymphomas (NHL) and Hodgkin lymphoma (HL).
- HL is the most common childhood cancer in the 15 to 19-year-old age group.
- Risk factors for Hodgkin lymphoma include geography, socio-economic factors, HIV infection, and family history.
- Early diagnosis of lymphoma greatly affects prognosis and treatment of the patient.
- Physician should introduce himself to the patient.
- Physician should know patient's name to establish good rapport with him.
- Physician should take history from the patient rather than other relatives.
- Permission for clinical examination from the patient is mandatory.
- Detailed history of patient's complain is an essential part of patient evaluation and without it physician might miss important and vital information.
- Proper clinical exam including GPE and focused examination as per patient complain is very important.
- Breaking bad news is an important skill that every physician should know.

- o Lymphoma and some malignancies can present in young patients especially if there is family history and other risk factors.
- o Social history including smoking history is essential.

*Abbreviation Elaboration

*GPE: General Physical Examination
*RA: Room Air
*PRN: Per Required Need

References

1. Thomas, J. and Monaghan, T. (2014). MPS selected chapters from the Oxford handbook of clinical examination and practical skills. Oxford: Oxford University Press.
2. Nicholas Joseph Talley and O'Connor, S. (2018). Talley & O'Connor's clinical examination. Chatswood, Nsw: Elsevier Australia.
3. www.uptodate.com. (n.d.). UpToDate. [online] Available at: https://www.uptodate.com/contents/clinical-presentation-and-diagnosis-of-classic-hodgkin-lymphoma-in-adults?search=hodgkin%20lymphoma&source=search_result&selectedTitle=2~150&usage_type=default&display_rank=2 [Accessed 4 Dec. 2021].
4. PDQ Adult Treatment Editorial Board (2002). Adult Hodgkin Lymphoma Treatment (PDQ®): Health Professional Version. [online] PubMed. Available at: https://www.ncbi.nlm.nih.gov/books/NBK66038/

Case Study 2

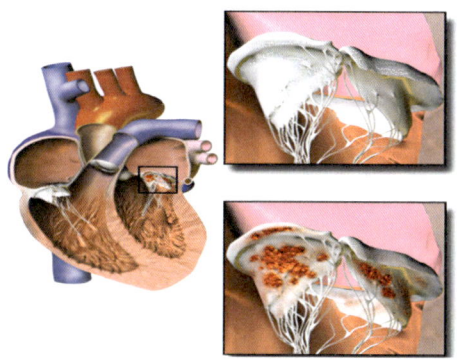

A 55-year-old female patient presented to Family Medicine Clinic complaining of fever from the last two weeks.

Physician: When did the fever start?
Patient: Two weeks.

Physician: Do you have other symptoms?
Patient: Yes, shortness of breath.

Physician: Do you have a cough?
Patient: No.
Physician examines chest by auscultation, no added sounds were found.

Physician: Okay, I think you have simple pneumonia, you need azithromycin for three days.

What went wrong in the previous scenario?

- Physician did not introduce himself.

- Physician did not ask the patient about her name to establish good rapport with her.
- Did not take permission for exam from the patient.
- Did not take detailed history of fever (degree of fever, nature of fever, response to antipyretics, associated symptoms including systematic review of all body systems).
- Did not take detailed history of shortness of breath (SOB) including aggravating and relieving factors, paroxysmal nocturnal dyspnea, orthopnea to differentiate between cardiac and non-cardiac causes of SOB.
- Did not ask about travel history, animal exposure, immunosuppression (with the degree noted), drug and toxin history which are essential in any patient presenting with fever.
- Did not do proper clinical exam especially cardiac and respiratory as patient complains of SOB.

Ideal Scenario

A 55-year-old female patient presented to Family Medicine Clinic complaining of fever for the last two weeks.

Physician: Asalam Alaykom. I am Dr. Ahmed. What is your name?
Patient: Saleha.

Physician: Salamat Saleha. What is your complaint?
Patient: I complain of fever.

Physician: For how long have you had fever?
Patient: For two weeks

Physician: Is it continuous or intermittent?
Patient: Continuous.

Physician: Did you measure it at home?
Patient: Yes.

Physician: How high is the fever?

Patient: 38^0 C.

Physician: Is it relieved by antipyretics?
Patient: No.

Physician: Is it more at a specific time in the day?
Patient: Yes, more at night during sleep.

Physician: Do you have previous episodes of the same complaint?
Patient: No.

Physician: Are there any aggravating or relieving factors?
Patient: No.

Physician: Do you have any chronic illnesses?
Patient: Yes, I have DM and HTN.

Physician: For how long do you have DM and HTN?
Patient: DM for 15 years and HTN for five years

Physician: Did you travel recently?
Patient: No.

Physician: Do you have an animal at home?
Patient: No.

Physician: Do you have other associated symptoms?
Patient: Yes, I have shortness of breath.

Physician: For how long do you have it?
Patient: One week.

Physician: Can you describe it?
Patient: I wake up from sleep with shortness of breath.

Physician: Do you have SOB once you lie on the bed?

Patient: No.

Physician: Do you have a cough or sputum?
Patient: No.

Physician: Do you have weight loss and lose appetite and night sweats?
Patient: No.

Physician: Have you underwent any surgery?
Patient: Yes, I change two heart valves with metallic ones.

Physician: When did you do it?
Patient: Six years ago.

Physician: What are your medications?
Patient: Glucophage, losartan and warfarin.

Physician: Okay Miss Saleha your complaint in summary. You are a 55 years old female, known case of DM and HTN, complaining of fever for the last 2 weeks continuously especially at night, associated with shortness of breath and Paroxysmal nocturnal dyspnea. You have a prosthetic heart valve done 6 years ago and you are taking Warfarin, Losartan and Glucophage.

Physician: Do you want to add any other information?
Patient: Yes…I have chills and rigor sometimes, also I have a headache.

Physician: Anything else you want to add?
Patient: Yes, I have a skin rash over my legs.

Physician: What is your concern Saleha?
Patient: I want you to investigate the reason for the fever.

Physician: What do you expect from me?
Patient: I want to know what my problem is.

During Examination:

Temperature: 39.3, pulse: 110b/min regular, BP: 99/70, O2 sat: 99% RA weight: 110 Kg, Height: 150 cm, GPE: patient looks ill.

Hand exam: there is reddish-brown lesions under the nail bed (Splinter hemorrhages)

There are also non-tender erythematous macules on the palms (Janeway lesions)

Legs: There is Petechial skin rash non-blanching non-palpable.

Heart Exam:

Inspection: There is sternal scar of previous CABG*.

Palpation: Apex beat palpable at fifth intercostal space with diffuse character.

Auscultation: Normal first and second heart sound with pansystolic murmur at apex radiating to left axilla.

Respiratory Exam:

Inspection: Same as in cardiac exam.

Palpation: Trachea in normal midline position with decrease chest expansion in both sides.

Percussion: Dullness over lung bases bilaterally.

Auscultation: There is reduced breath sounds at lung base in both sides with fine crackles in late respiration in both sides of chest mainly at lung bases.

Discussion and Counseling:

Physician: Okay, Miss Saleha, I think I have to do more investigation to know the diagnosis.

Patient: Okay, doctor.

Physician request basic labs including CBC, Biochemistry, CRP, ESR, chest X-ray, blood culture, sputum culture, urinalysis, ECG and ECHO.

Labs Results:

CBC showed leukocytosis (WBC: 25, HB: 9, plat 313).

Biochemistry: High CRP and ESR.

Blood culture: Preliminary result showed *Staphylococcus aureus*.

Chest Radiography: Bilateral pulmonary edema at lung bases bilaterally

ECG: Sinus tachycardia

ECHO: Movable mass with vegetation over mitral prosthetic valve with moderate mitral regurgitation.

(Patient came after doing the investigations.)

Patient: Doctor Ahmed, tell me about the investigations. I hope it will be good.

Physician: Yes! Saleha, please sit down. You know, Saleha, one of the complications of metallic heart valves is infection in the valve because the valve is a foreign body.

Patient: Yes, Doctor Ahmed, the surgeon told me about this.

Physician: Good! I think you have an infection in the heart valve causing valve regurgitation which is the reason for SOB.

Patient: Okay, what can I do now?

Physician: Do not worry. I will arrange for you everything because I am here to help you.

Patient: Thank you, doctor.

Physician: I will give you one dose of antibiotics here while I am arranging for you with the cardiology team.

Patient: I agree, doctor.

- Physician arranges for one dose of vancomycin in the infusion room after a test dose for allergy.
- Physician contacts cardiology service in the hospital and discuss with him the case and cardiology accept to see the patient as an emergency in the cardiology ward for admission.

Patient finished the dose of vancomycin.

Physician: Okay, Saleha. I arranged with the cardiology team just now to go to the cardiology ward. They will see you there and they will do the remaining work.

Patient: Thank you, Doctor Ahmed. You help me so much.

Physician: This is my job.
Patient: Thanks, Doctor Ahmed.

Physician: Do you have any questions?
Patient: No, thanks!

Physician checks the patient's understanding and gives her an appointment slip with cardiology.

Clinical Pearls and Take-Home Messages

- Early diagnosis significantly influences the outcome of patients with Endocarditis (IE), given its association with an invasive infection.
- Staphylococci, streptococci, and enterococci stand as the three most common global causes of IE.
- Clinical presentations of IE encompass fever, chills, anorexia, malaise, and headache. Additionally, the emergence of new or changing murmurs and signs of heart failure are crucial indicators.
- Supportive signs of infective endocarditis may manifest in cutaneous symptoms such as petechiae or splinter hemorrhages.
- Prosthetic valve endocarditis constitutes 20 percent of all IE cases, occurring in 1–6 percent of individuals with valve prostheses.

Definite IE is established in the presence of any of the following:	
Pathologic criteria	
Pathologic lesions – Vegetation or intracardiac abscess demonstrating active endocarditis on histology, **OR**	
Microorganism – Demonstrated by culture or histology of a vegetation or intracardiac abscess	
Clinical criteria	
Using specific definitions listed in **Table B**:	
2 major clinical criteria, **OR**	
1 major and 3 minor clinical criteria, **OR**	
5 minor clinical criteria	
Possible IE*	
Presence of 1 major and 1 minor clinical criteria **OR** presence of 3 minor clinical criteria	
Rejected IE	
A firm alternate diagnosis is made, **OR**	
Resolution of clinical manifestations occurs after ≤4 days of antibiotic therapy, **OR**	
No pathologic evidence of infective endocarditis is found at surgery or autopsy after antibiotic therapy for 4 days or less	
Clinical criteria for possible or definite IE not met	

Table 2: Modified Duke criteria for infective endocarditis

*Abbreviation Elaboration

CABG: Coronary Artery Bypass Graft

References

1. Chiefs, I.M. (n.d.). Chief's Corner: Infective Endocarditis. [online] Inside the Silver Fridge. Available at: https://www.thesilverfridge.com/blog/2018/7/13/chiefs-corner-infective-endocarditis.
2. Thomas, J. and Monaghan, T. (2020). Oxford handbook of clinical examination and practical skills. Oxford: Oxford University Press.
3. www.uptodate.com. (n.d.). UpToDate. [online] Available at:https://www.uptodate.com/contents/search?search=infective%20endocarditis&sp=0&searchType=PLAIN_TEXT&source=USER_INPUT&searchControl=TOP_PULLDOWN&s

Case Study 3

A 41-year-old woman presented with fever for three weeks…

Physician: Hello, my name is Dr. Ali. How can I help you?
Patient: I have fever for three weeks

Physician: Tell me more about your fever?
Patient: It Increases in the afternoon and responds to paracetamol.

Physician: Any abdominal pain or vomiting?
Patient: No.

Physician: Any upper respiratory tract symptoms?
Patient: No.

Physician: Any urine changes?
Patient: No.

Physician: Do you have a history of contact with sick person?
Patient: No.
Physician: Do you have any Past medical and surgical history?
Patient: I have history of cholecystectomy.

Examination:

Urinary dipstick: Unremarkable.

Investigation:

CBC, ESR, CRP, urine culture and blood culture.

Provisional Diagnosis:

Dengue fever

Plan:

- Amoxicillin/clavulanate dose 25-45 mg/kg Q12H for 7 days
- Follow up after 7 days

What went wrong in the previous scenario?

1. Travel history (a description of accommodations, information about pre-travel immunizations or chemoprophylaxis during travel, a sexual history, and a list of exposures and risk factors)
2. Contact with animals
3. Ingestion of raw or undercooked food
4. Unpasteurized milk
5. Proper investigation
6. Vital sign
7. Detailed history of fever
8. ICE (idea, concern, and expectation)
9. Prevention and education
10. Ask for senior help

Ideal Scenario

A 41 years old woman presented with fever for three weeks.

Physician: Hello, my name is Dr. Ali. How can I help you?
Patient: I have fever for three weeks

Physician: Tell me more about your fever?
Patient: It Increases in the afternoon and responds to paracetamol.

Physician: Do you have any night sweats?
Patient: Yes.

Physician: Any documented fever?

Patient: Yes, 39⁰ C at home that responds to paracetamol.
Physician: Any associated symptoms?
Patient: Fatigue, chills and rigors.

Physician: Any abdominal pain or vomiting?
Patient: Mild abdominal pain without vomiting.

Physician: Do you have diarrhea or constipation?
Patient: No.

Physician: Any upper respiratory tract symptoms?
Patient: No.
Physician: Any urinary changes?
Patient: No.

Physician: Any joint pain?
Patient: Yes, mainly in the early morning.

Physician: Any history of contact with sick persons?
Patient: No.

Physician: Any mosquito bites?
Patient: No.

Physician: Any weight loss or loss of appetite?
Patient: Yes, I lost 7 kg in the past three weeks.

Physician: Any history of travel?
Patient: Yes, I came back from Prague 1 month ago.

Physician: The reason for travel?
Patient: Vacation.

Physician: Where did you live?
Patient: In rural area with the local population.

Physician: Any ingestion of raw food or unpasteurized milk?
Patient: Yes, I ingested some unpasteurized milk in the whole trip.

Physician: Did you take vaccination or chemoprophylaxis before the trip?
Patient: No.
Physician: Do you have rash or animal scratch?
Patient: No
Physician: Sexual contact with new partner?

Patient: No.
Physician: ICE?

Patient:
Idea: prolonged fever due to serous disease.
Concern: That I have T.B.
Expectation: Proper investigation and treatment.

Physician: Any past medical and surgical history?
Patient: I have a history of C-section.

Examination:
- General: pale and sick
- Vital sign:
  - Temp: 39 C
  - Pulse 105b/m
  - RR: 15 b/m
  - Wt.: 70 kg
  - Ht.: 180 cm
  - BMI: 18.5
  - Skin: no rash
- Abdomen: hepato-splenomegaly
- L.N: generalized lymphadenopathy
- Chest: vesicular breath sounds + no added sound
- C.V.S: (S1+S2) first and second heart sounds are heard and there is no added sounds
- CNS: intact

- o ENT: normal

Investigation:

CBC (Leukocytosis, anemia, and thrombocytopenia).
Elevated ESR and CRP.
Liver enzyme, renal function, urine culture and blood culture.
Brucellosis antibody (titer more than 1:80).

Diagnosis:

Brucellosis

Treatment and Plan:

- o Start treatment with doxycycline 100 mg BID+ rifampin 600 mg OD for 6 weeks.
- o Supportive treatment with analgesic for pain and fever.
- o Referral to infectious disease.
- o Explain the side effects of the antibiotics.
- o Repeat brucella titer after completing treatment.

Prevention:

- o Avoid eating raw or undercooked meat.
- o Avoid unpasteurized dairy products.
- o Pre-traveler education, vaccination and chemoprophylaxis for the next trip.
- o Proper hand hygiene.

Differential Diagnosis:

- ❖ Cholera
- ❖ Non-typhoidal salmonellosis
- ❖ Trichinosis

- Typhoid fever
- Hepatitis A
- Tuberculosis
- Leptospirosis
- Schistosomiasis
- Dengue fever
- Malaria

Clinical Pearls and Take Home Messages

Guidelines for the evaluation of non-focal fever of travelers:

- Always consider common causes like urinary tract and upper respiratory infections.
- Keep in mind that the fever may be unrelated to recent travel, so explore non-travel-related factors.
- In cases with a short incubation period (less than 21 days), most patients likely have malaria, typhoid fever, or dengue fever.
- For cases with a prolonged incubation period (more than 21 days), consider malaria or tuberculosis as primary possibilities. Additionally, think about hepatitis A for unimmunized patients.
- Seek early consultation with an infectious diseases subspecialist if the patient is severely ill or has altered mental status.
- If following these guidelines doesn't lead to a diagnosis, explore uncommon causes and seek guidance from an infectious diseases specialist.
- Assess pre-travel immunizations and chemoprophylaxis used during travel.
- Practice preventive measures by avoiding undercooked meat and unpasteurized dairy products like milk, cheese, and ice cream.
- Individuals involved in hunting or handling animals should use protective gear such as rubber gloves, goggles, gowns, or aprons.
- In agricultural and meat processing work, implementing protective barriers and proper handling and disposal of afterbirths, animal carcasses, and internal organs is a vital prevention strategy.

References

1. Corbel, M. (1997). Brucellosis: an Overview. Emerging Infectious Diseases, 3(2), pp.213–221.
2. Anon, (2020). Prevention. [online] Available at: https://www.cdc.gov/brucellosis/prevention/index.html.
3. Humar, A. and Keystone, J. (1996). Fortnightly Review: Evaluating fever in travellers returning from tropical countries. BMJ, 312(7036), pp.953–956.
4. Anon, (2019). Treatment. [online] Available at: https://www.cdc.gov/brucellosis/treatment/index.html.

Case Study 4

25-year-old woman married with one child presented with fever, lower abdominal pain and unusual vaginal discharge.

Physician: For how long have you had your fever?
Patient: For four days, on and off respond to paracetamol.

Physician: Can you describe your abdominal pain?
Patient: Lower abdominal pain radiating to the back.

Physician: Describe your vaginal discharge.
Patient: Heavy discharge, foul smelling and greenish in color.

Physician: Is there any urinary symptoms?
Patient: Yes

Physician: UDS (urine dipstick): leukocyte 2+
Others: normal

Provisional diagnosis: Bacterial vaginitis

Plan:

Metronidazole 500 mg 2 times a day for 7 days
Discharge the patient

What went wrong in the previous scenario?

1. Introduce yourself.
2. Open ended question.

3. Detailed history about (last menstrual period, contraception method, sexual history).
4. No examination done.
5. More investigation need to be done.
6. Didn't ask about ICE (idea, concern and expectation).
7. Screening for depression and smoking.
8. Past medical and surgical history.
9. Didn't involve the patient in the treatment plan.

Ideal Scenario

25-year-old woman married with one child presented with fever, lower abdominal pain and unusual vaginal discharge.

Physician: Any aggravating or relieving factor?
Patient: Aggravated by intercourse and relieved by painkillers.

Physician: Are you on any contraception?
Patient: Yes, IUD (intrauterine device).

Physician: When it was inserted?
Patient: Three weeks ago, in the OBGYN clinic.

Physician: Any prophylactic medication was given?
Patient: No.

Physician: Do you experience any dyspareunia?
Patient: Yes, I did the last 2 weeks.

Physician: Tell me when it was your last menstrual bleeding?
Patient: Three weeks ago.

Physician: Is there any postcoital bleeding?
Patient: Yes, lately 2 times happened.

Physician: ICE?
Patient: Idea: IUD causing some kind of infection.

Concern: Do I need surgery?
Expectation: Treatment or IUD removal.

Physician: How is your mood and interest?
Patient: My mood and interest are good.

Physician: Any past medical or surgical history?
Patient: No.

Physician: Any past OBGYN history?
Patient: No.

Examination:

- General: pale
- Vital sign:
  - Temp: 38.5 C
  - Pulse: 90 B/M
  - RR: 13 B/m
  - BMI: 23
- UDS: leukocyte 2+

Blood: 2+
Others: normal

- Abdomen: mild lower abdominal tenderness, no rebound
- Vaginal examination: Cervical motion tenderness

Investigation:

Urine analysis and culture
Blood test: CBC (leukocytosis), elevated CRP, and ESR
Vaginal swab and pap smear
Pregnancy test

Ultrasound scan

Diagnosis:

PID (pelvic inflammatory disease)

Treatment:

Ceftriaxone 250 mg IM plus Doxycycline 100 mg twice per day for 14 days

Plan:

- OBGYN referral in case you didn't respond to treatment in the next 72 hours.
- If the pain and fever didn't improve come back.
- Follow up after 2 days.

IUD shouldn't be removed unless you didn't respond to treatment within 48-72 hours

Physician: Do you have any questions?
Patient: Yes, what about my fertility is there any effect on it?

Physician: Based on the history and examination the answer is no.

Differential diagnosis:

- Cervicitis
- UTI
- Appendicitis
- Endometriosis
- Ovarian torsion
- Interstitial cystitis
- Tubo-ovarian abscess
- Less commonly ovarian tumor

Clinical Pearls and Take-Home Messages

Intrauterine devices (IUDs) do not pose an increased risk for pelvic inflammatory disease (PID) beyond the initial 20 days post-insertion.

IUDs do not require removal if the patient shows clinical improvement within 48 to 72 hours of starting antibiotics.

While there is no specific screening recommendation for PID, testing for chlamydia and gonorrhea has proven to reduce PID incidence in high-risk populations.

The American College of Obstetricians and Gynecologists does not advise prophylactic antibiotics for procedures like colposcopy, loop electrosurgical excision, endometrial biopsy, IUD insertion, or endometrial ablation.

Antibiotic prophylaxis is recommended for women undergoing hysterosalpingography if they have a history of PID or dilated tubes during the procedure. It is also recommended for uterine evacuation in early pregnancy loss and first or second-trimester abortions.

Supplemental Criteria to Increase the Specificity of a Pelvic Inflammatory Disease Diagnosis

Cervical mucopurulent discharge or friability

Elevated C-reactive protein

Elevated erythrocyte sedimentation rate

Large number* of white blood cells on saline microscopy of vaginal fluid

Oral temperature greater than 101°F (38.3°C)

Testing positive for *Neisseria gonorrhoeae* or *Chlamydia trachomatis*

Table 3: Supplemental Criteria to assist in diagnosing Pelvic inflammatory Disease

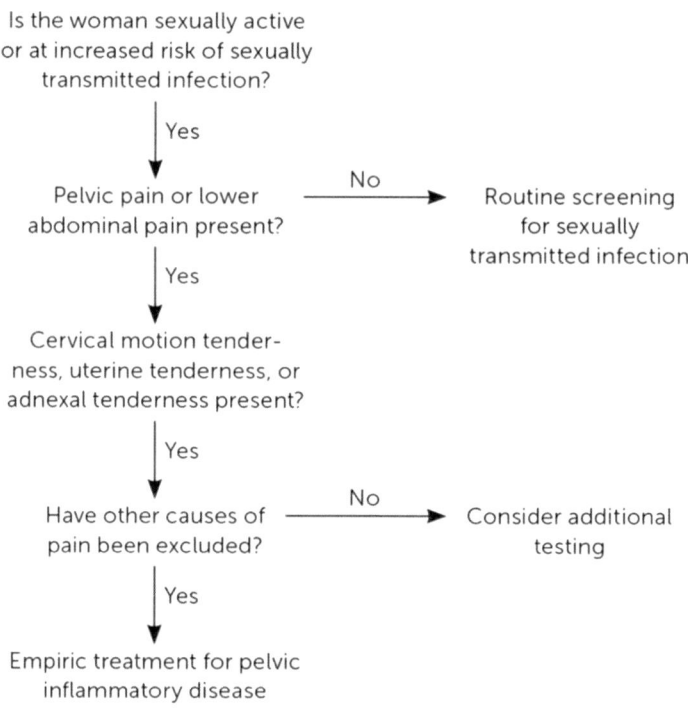

Figure 1: Female pelvic pain investigation pathway

References

1. www.cdc.gov. (2021). Bacterial Vaginosis – STI Treatment Guidelines. [online] Available at: https://www.cdc.gov/std/treatment-guidelines/bv.htm.
2. Mayoclinic.org. (2018). Pelvic inflammatory disease (PID) – Diagnosis and treatment – Mayo Clinic. [online] Available at: https://www.mayoclinic.org/diseases-conditions/pelvic-inflammatory-disease/diagnosis-treatment/drc-20352600.
3. www.cdc.gov. (2021). Pelvic Inflammatory Disease (PID) – STI Treatment Guidelines. [online] Available at: https://www.cdc.gov/std/treatment-guidelines/pid.htm.
4. Grimes, D.A. (2000). Intrauterine device and upper-genital-tract infection. The Lancet, 356(9234), pp.1013–1019.

Back Pain Chapter

AHMAD A. ALGARNI, MD
FATEN F. RAGAB, MD
OMAR S. ALZAHRANI, MD

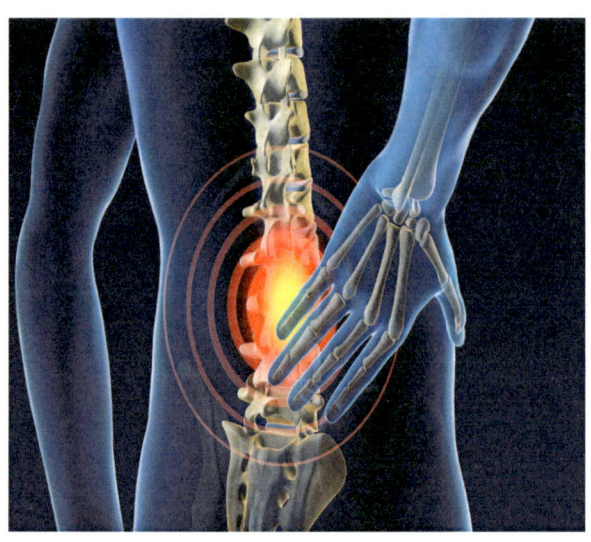

Case Study 1

A 39-year-old male patient, married with three kids, not known to have any medical problem. He came to the Family Medicine Clinic complaining of back pain.

Physician: For how long do you have back pain?
Patient: For five years.

Physician: Is it radiating to the lower limb?
Patient: No.

Physician: Do you have any relieving or aggravating factors?
Patient: No.

Physician: Any labs or X-rays done before?
Patient: I visited many doctors during this period including G. Ps*, orthopedics and neurosurgeons, many labs and radiological studies including lumbar MRI, but they told me, "You have no problem."

Physician: Most likely you have muscular strain and you need only analgesics.
Physician prescribes paracetamol and diclofenac gel and discharge the patient from the clinic.

Mistakes:
Doctor used a closed ended question.
Doctor did not establish a good rapport with the patient.
Doctor did not ask about ICE (idea, concern, expectation).
Doctor did not ask about social issues.

There is no screening for depression.
Doctor did not examine the patient.

Ideal Scenario

A 39 years old male patient, married with three kids, not known to have any medical problem. He came to the Family Medicine Clinic complaining of back pain.

Physician: Welcome to my clinic! My name is Dr.Ahmad, and I'm happy to help you.
Patient: Thank you, Dr. Ahmad.

Physician: Can you tell me more about your pain?
Patient: I started complaining of back pain more than five years back. This pain is moderate in severity, aching in nature, and diffuse in my lower back.

Physician: Okay, can you give me information about relieving, aggravating and associated symptoms?
Patient: I did not have any aggravating or relieving factors and was not associated with any symptoms and not spreading in any other parts of my body.

Physician: Okay, can you give your ideas and concerns about your problem?
Patient: I don't know, but I visited many doctors during this period including G. Ps, orthopedics, and neurosurgeons, many labs and radiological studies including lumbar MRI were done, but they told me, "You have no problem." I received different analgesia without any improvement.

At the end of the complaint, he told the doctor that nobody believes him.

Physician: What about your expectations from me?
Patient: Please Dr. Ahmad I feel so tired and need to rest for a while.

Dr. Ahmad noticed that he has depressive mode, so he asked him about other symptoms of depression like pleasures and interests in his life, and he found the patient has most of the criteria of major depression. On examination, he has a normal gait. There were no deformities of the back. No muscle rigidity. No tenderness or other abnormalities with intact motor and sensory functions of his lower limb.

And diagnosed the patient with Somatic symptom disorder with comorbid depression and he started analgesic and antidepressant medication.

And he informs the patient that improvement of his symptoms can depend on how much he alters his lifestyle and that it is his responsibility to do this. Common problems include poor sleep patterns, inability to set limits on personal goals and on demands from other people, lack of assertiveness, inadequate social skills, and inability to set priorities in life. The patient should be encouraged to seek professional help when needed.

Clinical Pearls and Take-Home Messages

- The doctor must be nonjudgmental, respectful, and empathetic. Listening with patience is more important than attempting to provide a quick solution.
- He needs to establish a supportive relationship. Inform patients that these symptoms tend to run a long course and may fluctuate according to changing psychosocial situations.
- Treatment of coexisting psychiatric disorders (depression).
- He needs to provide medications for supportive treatment, such as analgesics for pain and other medications if needed. These prescriptions are needed for symptom relief and as a sign of acceptance of the symptoms. Antidepressants may be effective for treating Somatic symptom disorders even when there is no coexisting depressive disorder.
- He needs to allow the patient to participate in decisions regarding the choice of treatment.
- He needs to encourage rehabilitation treatment, including exercise, physical therapy, yoga, and participation in social activities.
- To inform the patient that improvement of their symptoms can depend on how much he alters his lifestyle and that it is his responsibility to do this. Common problems include poor sleep patterns, inability to set limits on personal goals and on demands from other people, lack of assertiveness, inadequate social skills, and inability to set priorities in life. The patient should be encouraged to seek professional help when needed.
- To explore relationships in the patient's family and at work and whether significant life events have occurred.

- To look for possible relationships between what is happening in the patients 'lives and his symptoms and help him see the connection.
- To refer the patient for psychological intervention to address their current life events as well as interpersonal conflicts.

*Abbreviation Elaboration

*GP: General Practitioner

References

1. Hall-flavin (2019). Depression can cause pain – and pain can cause depression. [online] Mayo Clinic. Available at: https://www.mayoclinic.org/diseases-conditions/depression/expert-answers/pain-and-depression/faq-20057823.
2. Kurlansik, S.L. and Maffei, M.S. (2016). Somatic Symptom Disorder. American Family Physician, [online] 93(1), pp.49–54. Available at: https://www.aafp.org/afp/2016/0101/p49.html.

Case Study 2

A 65 years old male patient with a known case of DM and HTN, on regular follow up.

He came to his family physician with lower back pain for more than four months, but he did not seek medical advice because his pain was mild. In the last week, the pain gradually increased in severity.

Physician: How do you feel your pain?
Patient: It is aching, doctor.

Physician: On a scale of 0-10, how severe is the pain, if zero is no pain and ten is the worst pain you have ever experienced?
Patient: It is about 7/10.

Physician: Is it continuous or interrupted?
Patient: It is all the time.

Physician: Do you notice anything that makes your pain more or less?
Patient: I noticed when I walk or sit or even stand the pain increases in its severity, but some are relieved with rest and the use of over-the-counter analgesia.

Physician: Is the pain going to other areas?
Patient: No, doctor.

Physician: Do you feel any weakness or changes in the sensation of your lower limbs?
Patient: No, doctor.

Physician: Do you have any other symptoms like urine or fecal incontinence?

Patient: No, doctor.

After that, the doctor started to examine the patient. He found mild to moderate tenderness with muscle spasms over the lumbar vertebrae and left sacroiliac joint pain.

Physician: No problem, I will do some investigations and x-rays on your back to see what is wrong. I will schedule your appointment after two weeks plus Tramal to control your pain.

Mistakes

The doctor did a great job to find the cause of the problem, but he needs to ask more questions which will help him to reach the diagnosis which includes the following:

- Medication history
- Allergic history
- Family history
- Traveling history
- Trauma history
- Associated symptoms and red flags (hematuria, weight loss, loss of appetite, generalized weakness, fever and morning stiffness)

Ideal Scenario

Physician: How do you feel your pain?
Patient: It is aching, doctor.

Physician: On a scale of 0-10, how severe is the pain, if zero is no pain and ten is the worst pain you have ever experienced?
Patient: It is about 7/10.

Physician: Is it continuous or interrupted?
Patient: It is all the time.

Physician: Do you notice anything that makes your pain more or less?

Patient: I noticed when I walk or sit or even stand the pain increase in its severity, but some are relieved with rest and the use of over-the-counter analgesia.

Physician: Is the pain going to other areas?
Patient: No, Doctor.

Physician: Do you feel any weakness or changes in the sensation of your lower limbs?
Patient: No, Doctor.

Physician: Do you have any other symptoms like urine or fecal incontinence?
Patient: No, Doctor.

Physician: Do you have any of these symptoms (fever, hematuria, weight loss, and generalized weakness)?
Patient: Actually, I have only loss of weight (about 10kg in 2months), and generalized weakness.

Physician took full medical, surgical, travel, social and psychological history.

After that, the doctor started to examine the patient. He found mild to moderate tenderness with muscle spasms over the lumbar vertebrae and left sacroiliac joint pain.

Physician: No problem, I will do some investigations and x-rays on your back to see what is wrong. I will schedule your appointment within days plus Tramal to control your pain.

In the next visit, the patient came to his G.P again and the doctor asks the patient about his pain, and he reported significant improvement regarding pain especially after starting Tramal.

The x-ray findings: Osteoplastic changes in the whole lumbar vertebrae and in the left sacroiliac joint which goes with metastasis from prostate adenocarcinoma that needs further workup.

Lab Investigations:
High PSA*.

The management:

So, the physician did an urgent referral to the urologist for further workup and management especially since the patient has the risk of cord compression.

Clinical Pearls and Take-Home Messages

Family physician should screen for red flags which include;

- Progressive motor or sensory loss, new urinary retention or overflow incontinence or new fecal incontinence
- Significant trauma relative to age
- Prolonged corticosteroid use
- Age older than 70 years, osteoporosis
- Spinal procedures in the past 12 months
- Intravenous drug use, immunosuppression, distant lumbar spine surgery
- History of metastatic cancer
- Unexplained weight loss
- Saddle anesthesia, loss of anal sphincter tone, significant motor deficits encompassing multiple nerve roots
- Contusions or abrasions
- Fever, wound in the spinal region
- Localized pain and tenderness
- Focal tenderness and localized pain in the setting of risk factors

*Abbreviations Elaborations

*PSA: Prostate Specific Antigen

References

1. Ziu, E., Viswanathan, V.K. and Mesfin, F.B. (2020). Cancer, Spinal Metastasis. [online] PubMed. Available at: https://www.ncbi.nlm.nih.gov/books/NBK441950/.
2. https://www.mayoclinicproceedings.org/article/S0025-6196(11)61965-4/fulltext

Case Study 3

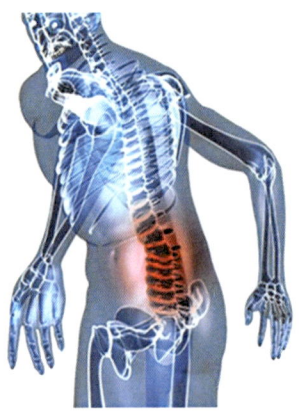 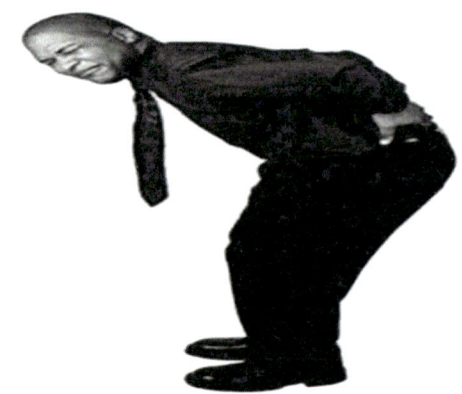

A 25-year-old male, accountant in a big bank, single came to the Family Medicine Clinic. The patient was complaining of low back pain.

Physician: When did your pain start?
Patient: Four days ago.

Physician: Did you have any history of trauma?
Patient: No.

Physician: Okay, Mr. Mohammed. I think you have a problem with your back, So you can go now to do a plain X-ray. Then, you can come after 1 week to check the results.

Mistakes:

- The physician did not introduce himself to the patient.
- Did not establish a good rapport with the patient.

- Did not ask detailed history about the pain, site, duration, character, severity in scale from 1–10, aggravating and relieving factors, radiation and associated symptoms.
- Did not ask the patient about the nature of his work.
- Early judgment of the cause of pain and the diagnosis.
- Did not ask about the patient ICE (idea, concern and expectation).
- Did not do clinical examination for the patient.
- Did not share the patient in the management plan.
- Did not discharge the patient on any relieving pain treatment.

Ideal Scenario

A 25 years old male, accountant in a big Bank, coming to the Family Medicine Clinic. Was complaining of low back pain.

Physician: Welcome Mr. Mohammed! My name is Dr. Mona, how can I help you?
Patient: Welcome Dr. Mona, I have low back pain.

Physician: For how long Mr. Mohammed?
Patient: For almost four days doctor.

Physician: Would you please tell me more about this pain?
Patient: I have low back pain for four days now and I cannot walk or sit as usual because of the pain.

Physician: What does the pain looks like?
Patient: It is a deep steady ache.

Physician: Is there anything that increases or decreases this pain?
Patient: Usually the pain increases at night and during movements.

Physician: Are there any associated symptoms?
Patient: No.

Physician: Can you tell me more about the nature of your work?

Patient: I am working as an accountant in a big bank. I am working for 9 hours per day, sitting most of the time in front of my computer and when I go home usually, I spend another four hours in front of the computer studying as I am preparing for Master Degree in Finance.

Physician: Did you have any history of trauma?
Patient: No.

Physician: Did you try any painkillers?
Patient: Yes, I tried paracetamol that decreases the pain slightly for some times and then the pain comes back.

Physician: On a scale from 1 to 10, can you rate the severity of pain?
Patient: In most of the time it is 5 out of 10.

Physician: Does the pain go down to your legs?
Patient: No.

Physician: Do you feel any tingling sensations or numbness of your legs?
Patient: No.

Physician: Are you controlling your bowel Mr. Mohammed?
Patient: Yes.

Physician: Do you feel any increase in your body temperature?
Patient: No.
Physician: Do you have any history of chronic illness?
Patient: No.

Physician: Did you undergo any previous surgeries before?
Patient: No.

Physician: Do you have any family history of the same condition?
Patient: No.

Physician: What about your mood and interest in life?

Patient: I am fine doctor, enjoying life with my family and preparing to get married next month.

Physician: Are you doing any sort of exercise?
Patient: No.

Physician: Are you a smoker?
Patient: Yes, I smoke one pack per day for almost five years.

Physician: Does the pain disturb your sleep or you wake up in the morning suffering of the pain?
Patient: No.

Physician: Do you have any history of weight loss?
Patient: No.

Physician: Any history of recent travel?
Patient: No.

Physician: Okay, Mr. Mohammed let me summarize your condition. You are 25 years old, accountant and preparing for master degree, sitting at least 13 hours per day in front of the computer, not doing any sort of exercise, smoker for 5 years and you have low back pain for four days without any history of trauma, pain increases at night, with movement and it does not disturb your sleep, no associated fever, no weight loss, no loss of bowel control.

Physician: Do you want to add anything else?
Patient: No.

Physician: Do you have any idea or concern about the cause of your back pain?
Patient: Maybe because I have disc, my friend has disc and he is feeling the same pain.

Physician: What do you expect from me?
Patient: I need something to relieve my pain and to get relief.

Physician: Okay, Mr. Mohammed can I examine you, please?

On Examination:

- Patient is vitally stable:
- temperature: 37 °C
- Pulse 84 per minute, regular
- BP 130/80
- Oxygen sat 100%
- Weight 90 kg
- Height 169 cm
- BMI=31.5.
- Gait is normal but slow because of the pain.
- Back exam:

- Inspection: patient is sitting on the edge of the chair, tilting to the left side.
- Palpation: normal spinal curvature, both shoulders are symmetrical, both hips are on the same line, tenderness at right paraspinal muscle at lumber area with moderate stiffness.
- Movement: freely mobile with tenderness elicited on flexion, extension and rotation of the back to the right side.
- Special tests: negative straight leg raising (SST) and femoral stretch test (FST).
- Muscle power of the lower extremities: 5/5.
- Neuro vascular examination: Sensation and pulsation of the lower limb are preserved.

Discussion and Counselling:

Physician: Okay Mr. Mohammed, after taking history and examining you, I don't think that you have any disc disorder like your friend. I think you have muscle strain that causes mechanical low back pain in our medical terms which is usually positional due to bad posture, you are sitting too much in front of the computer without any activities.

Also, you have increased weight, you have obesity together with smoking that need another medical care.

Patient: So, what can you offer me doctor, I tried to lose weight myself many times. I also tried to quit smoking but I failed.

Physician: Okay Mr. Mohammed let us discuss your problems one by one.

First regarding your back pain, since you don't have any warning symptoms and signs you can use painkillers together with muscle relaxant. Your pain will diminish within six weeks or before.

Second, we should pay attention to your weight and smoking. Our hospital can offer you extra care through lifestyle modification clinic and smoking cessation clinic that will help you in these two issues.

We will reassess you after 6 weeks. If you are not improving, your pain is worsening and goes down to your legs, or any numbness of your legs during this period, please come at any time and we can refer you to spinal surgery. And I want to advise you to use ice and hot compresses several times per day for 15-20 minutes. Being active can help you get up – and slowly start moving back again.

Stretching is good practice, walking, yoga and swimming are also good exercises that can help maintain the flexibility of muscles and other tissues while the sprain recovers. Don't sit for long times. Try to move every 30 minutes.

Physician: Do you want to ask me any question Mr. Mohammed?
Patient: Thank you, Dr. Mona.

Clinical Pearls and Take-Home Messages

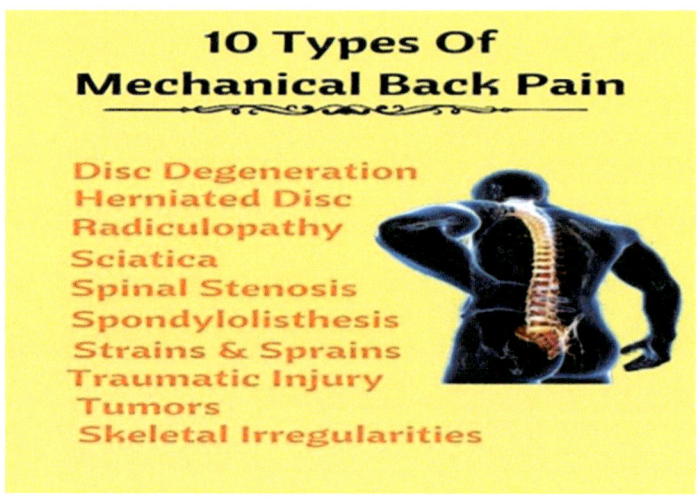

Table 4: Common types of Mechanical Back pain

How Can Low Back Pain Develop?

Trauma, whether major or minor, is a significant factor contributing to back pain. Identifying major trauma is straightforward, encompassing incidents like slips, falls, sports injuries, or car accidents. On the other hand, minor traumas, often repetitive in nature such as overuse injuries, are more challenging to pinpoint. These minor traumas involve physical movements, postures, and loads on the spine that led to tissue damage, eventually resulting in pain, especially in the case of low back pain.

Sprains and strains are widely considered the most common causes of back pain, particularly in acute episodes that self-resolve. Strains involve injuries to muscles or their connecting tendons, while sprains affect ligaments connecting bones. A sedentary lifestyle is recognized as a potential contributor to various health issues, including back pain, leading to the assertion that "Sitting is the new smoking."

Incorrect movement and posture patterns, such as lifting improperly, excessive bending and twisting, using a too-soft mattress or pillow, prolonged periods of sitting, standing, or driving, and poor office work habits, can also contribute to back pain.

Differential Diagnosis of Mechanical Low Back Pain

Diagnosis (percentage of patients with low back pain)	Key characteristics and clinical clues
Lumbosacral muscle strains/sprains (70%)	Often following isolated traumatic incidents or repetitive overuse; pain worse with movement, relieved by rest; examination may reveal restricted range of motion, muscle tenderness, or trigger points
Lumbar spondylosis (10%)	More common in persons older than 40 years; pain may be present in or radiate from the hips; pain is worse with activity; pain may worsen with lumbar spine extension or rotation; neurologic examination is usually normal
Disk herniation (5% to 10%)	Most often involves the L5 or S1 nerve root, at L4-L5 or L5-S1 in 90% to 95% of cases; symptoms may include pain, paresthesia, sensory change, loss of strength or reflexes depending on affected nerve root
Spondylolysis (less than 5%*)	Common in young athletes; symptoms often develop insidiously; pain with activities involving lumbar extension; imaging is diagnostic, but early imaging in the absence of red flags is typically not necessary; usually occurs in a lower lumbar vertebra, most often L5
Vertebral compression fracture (4%)	Fracture may occur slowly over time or acutely with mild trauma; acute episodes usually resolve in four to six weeks, but abnormal healing or additional fractures may result in chronic pain and functional impairment; presents as localized back pain that is worse with flexion and often point tenderness on palpation; risk factors include increased age, history of trauma, chronic steroid use, and osteoporosis; plain radiography should be obtained to confirm diagnosis
Spondylolisthesis (3% to 4%)	Pain often radiates into the buttocks or posterior thigh; leg pain may be worse than back pain; often presents as paresthesias, numbness, or weakness; occurs at L5 in 90% of cases
Spinal stenosis (3%)	Presents as back pain, sometimes with sensory loss or weakness in the legs; calf pain with ambulation that is relieved with rest/sitting (pseudoclaudication); neurologic examination findings are normal; imaging is diagnostic

*—Occurs in less than 5% of the general population but in up to 50% of preadolescent and adolescent athletes.

Information from references 1 through 3, 5 through 7, and 11.

Table 5: Differential diagnosis of mechanical low back pain
American Academy of Family Physician

- ➢ Home message to family physician:
- Physician should introduce himself to the patient.
- Show empathy and try to make good rapport with the patient.
- Take full detailed history.
- Ask open ended questions.
- Don't be judgmental.
- Let the patient explore his idea, concern and expectations.
- Don't skip focused examination.

- Treat the patient as a whole and don't miss his/her daily habits and life style especially in young patients.
- Don't ignore the patient's psychology.
- Always remember management should be patient centered meaning that you should share the patient with every single step in your management plan.
- Don't forget to alert the patient about the red flags.
- Don't forget that most of the muscle problems are due to overuse.
- Don't ignore asking about the patient's social life, sometimes it is a clue to solve the patient's condition.

References

1. National Clinical Guidelines for non-surgical treatment of patients with recent onset low back pain or lumbar radiculopathy. Stochkendahl MJ, Kjaer P, Hartvigsen J, et al. Eur Spine J 2018; 27: 60-75.
2. American Academy of Family Physician (AAFP).
3. Low back pain and radicular pain: assessment and management. KCE report 287Cs. Brussels: Belgian Health Care Knowledge Centre (KCE),Van Wambeke P, Desomer A, Ailliet L, et al. Summary: 2017.
4. Noninvasive treatments for acute, subacute, and chronic low back pain: a clinical practice guideline from the American College of Physicians. Qaseem A, Wilt TJ, McLean RM, et al. Ann Intern Med 2017; 166: 514-530. 2017.

Case Study 4

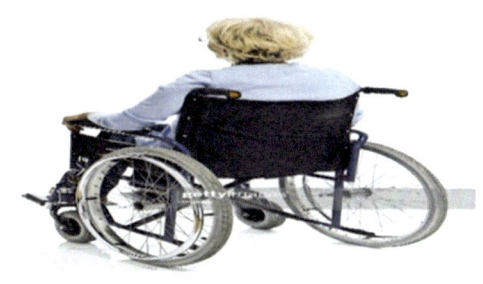

A 70-year-old female, house wife, mother of seven sons coming to Family Medicine on a wheelchair with her oldest son. The patient was complaining of severe low back pain.

Physician: When did your pain start?
Patient: One week ago.

Physician: Why are you coming on a wheelchair? Do you have any problem with your legs?
Patient: Because of my back pain.

Physician: Did you have any history of trauma?
Patient: I don't remember.
The son: Excuse me doctor, last week, we found her on the floor while she was going to the toilet. She fell down.

Physician to the relative: Did you take her to any hospital then?
The son: No, I was at work and my wife told me that she fell down on her back while going to the toilet.

Physician: Okay, I think your pain is due to the falling down. I will write a pain killer local and tablet, and you will be fine.

Mistakes:
- The physician did not introduce himself to the patient.
- Did not establish a good rapport with the patient.
- Did not ask for a detailed history about the pain, site, duration, character of pain, severity in scale from 1-10, aggravating and relieving factors, radiation and associated symptoms.
- Did not ask about her co-morbidities and her daily medications.
- Early judgment of the cause of pain and the diagnosis.
- Did not ask about the patient ICE (idea, concern and expectation).
- Did not do clinical examination for the patient.
- Did not share the patient in the plan of management.
- Did not explore about the cause of falling down, and if it is for the first time or recurrent.

Ideal Scenario

A 70-year-old female, house wife, mother of seven sons, coming to Family Medicine Clinic on a wheelchair together with her eldest son complaining of low back pain.

Physician: Welcome, Mom Salha! My name is Dr. Faten, how can I help you?
Patient: How are you, Dr. Faten? I have severe low back pain.

Physician: For how long, Mom Salha?
Patient: For almost one week doctor.

Physician: Would you please tell me more about this pain?
Patient: I had low back pain for almost 1 year, but the pain became so severe one week ago, I cannot walk as usual because of the pain.

Physician: Is there anything that increases or decreases this pain?
Patient: Usually the pain increases when I lie down.
Physician: Are there any associated symptoms?
Patient: No.

Physician: Did you try any painkillers?
Patient: Yes, I tried paracetamol that decreases the pain slightly for some times and then the pain comes back.

Physician: On a scale from 1 to 10, can you rate the severity of pain?
Patient: Most of the time it is 7 out of 10.

Physician: Does the pain go down to your legs?
Patient: No.

Physician: Do you feel any tingling sensation or numbness of your legs?
Patient: No

Physician: Did you have any history of trauma?
Patient: I don't remember.
The son: Excuse me doctor, my wife told me that my mother felt down one week ago on her back while going to the toilet. She was dizzy, but didn't lose her consciousness. My wife checked her blood sugar, and it was low. She gave her some sweets.

Physician: Is it the first time to have low blood sugar, sir?
Son: Recently, she has recurrent low blood sugar. She is not eating well.

Physician: Are you controlling your bowel, Mom Salha?
Patient: Yes, to some extent but this is my problem for years with my urine control.

Physician: Do you feel any increase in your body temperature?
Patient: No.

Physician: Do you have any history of chronic illnesses?
Patient: Yes, Dr. Faten. I have diabetes, high blood pressure, high cholesterol and osteoporosis.

Physician: What medication are you taking, Mom Salha?
Patient: Here is my medications, Dr. Faten.

The doctor opens her medicine box, it contains Insulin pens, Amlodipine, Atorvastatin, Perindopril, Alendronate, Calcium and Vitamin D.

Physician: Who are taking care of you, Mom Salha?
Patient: My son and his wife.

Physician: Did you undergo any previous surgeries before?
Patient: No.

Physician: What about your mood and interest in life?
Patient: I am fine doctor. I am enjoying life with my family, but now I am in pain.

Physician: Okay, Mom Salha, let me summarize your condition, you are 70 years old, house wife, mother of 7 sons, known case of diabetes, high blood pressure, high cholesterol and osteoporosis, on insulin + Amlodipine + Atorvastatin +Alendronate +Vitamin D +Calcium and Coversyl. You came today complaining of low back pain for one year that is increasing for one week after falling down on your back, no numbness of the extremities, no radiation of pain, no increase in your body temperature and you are controlling your bowel to some extent.
Physician: Do you want to add anything else?
Patient: No.

Physician: Do you have any ideas about the cause of your back pain?
Patient: Maybe, because I felt down on my back or something else.

Physician: Any concerns?
Patient: I am afraid. Maybe, I have brucellosis like my sister.

Physician: What do you expect from me?
Patient: I need something to relieve my pain.

Physician: Okay, Mom Salha. I will examine you. Please, do not worry. I will support you.

On Examination:

- Patient is vitally stable: temperature: 36.9 c, pulse 80 per minute, regular, BP=135/70. Oxygen sat 100%, weight 60 kg, height 155 cm, BMI=25, pain scale 7/10, RBS*=180 mg/dl
- gait is normal
- Back exam:
  ❖ Inspection: there is some kyphosis at the upper back, ecchymotic patch at the lumbar spine area.

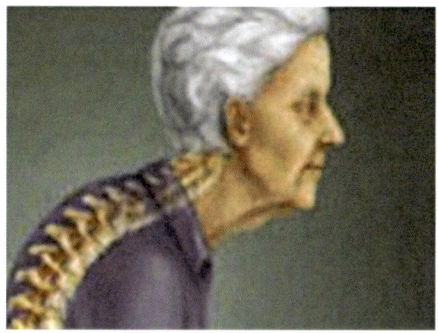

Figure 2: Kyphosis of the upper spine

❖ Palpation: tenderness at upper part of lumbar spine
❖ Movement: freely mobile with tenderness elicited on flexion, extension and rotation of the back
❖ Special tests: negative SST and FST
❖ Muscle power of the lower extremities: 5/5
❖ Sensation and pulsation of the lower limb are preserved

Discussion and Counselling:

Physician: Okay, Mom Salha, after taking history and examining you, I don't think that you have brucellosis like your sister, but may be something in your spine. Do you mind if we do a plain x ray for your back to confirm my diagnosis?

Patient: No, Dr. Faten. I am ready to do the X-ray.

Physician: Mom Salha, the X-ray image shows that you have thinning of the bone in your spine due to osteoporosis which causes compression of the vertebra at your lower back. We call it compression fracture.

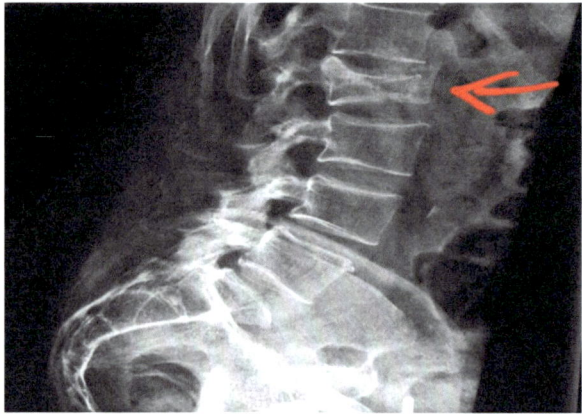

Figure 3: later Lumbosacral x ray showing Lumber compression Fracture (Arrow)

Patient: Is it serious Doctor? Can I walk normally later on? What can you do for me?

Physician: Don't worry, Mom Salha. We will take care of you. Do you mind if we start giving you painkiller tablets one tablet every twelve hours and a local gel. You can put it on the painful area of your back three times per day, and I will arrange appointment with our physiotherapist. Usually the condition heels after 8 to 12 weeks.

We will reassess you after 12 weeks. If you are not improving or if you find your pain is worsening, the pain goes down to your legs, or you feel any numbness of your legs during this period, please come at any time. We can refer you to spinal surgery.

And I want to advice you for using walking aids, gradual mobilization, and I think you need to take care of your blood sugar, so I can make an appointment for you with the chronic illness clinic.

Patient: Thank you, Dr. Faten.

Clinical Pearls and Take-Home Messages

Vertebral compression fractures (VCFs) stand as the most prevalent complication of osteoporosis, and the risk of fractures escalates with age. Four out of ten white women over 50 years are expected to experience a hip, spine, or vertebral fracture during their lifetime.

VCFs can result in chronic pain, disfigurement, height loss, limitations in daily activities, heightened risk of pressure sores, pneumonia, and psychological distress. Patients with an acute VCF may describe sudden back pain triggered by position changes, coughing, sneezing, or lifting. While physical examination findings are often normal, kyphosis and midline spine tenderness may be observed. More than two-thirds of patients are asymptomatic and incidentally diagnosed through plain radiography. Analgesics like acetaminophen, non-steroidal anti-inflammatory drugs, narcotics, and calcitonin are among the treatments for acute VCFs. However, physicians must consider potential adverse effects, especially in older patients. Conservative therapeutic options involve limited bed rest, bracing, physical therapy, nerve root blocks, and epidural injections. Percutaneous vertebral augmentation, such as vertebroplasty and kyphoplasty, remains controversial but can be considered for patients with insufficient pain relief from nonsurgical approaches or when persistent pain significantly impacts quality of life. Family physicians play a crucial role in preventing vertebral fractures by managing risk factors and addressing osteoporosis.

Home Message to Family Physician

- Physician should introduce himself to the patient.
- Show empathy and try to make good rapport with the patient.
- Take full detailed history.
- Ask open ended questions.
- Don't be judgmental.
- Let the patient explore his idea, concern and expectation.
- Don't skip focused examination.
- Treat the patient as a whole and put his co morbidities and his poly-pharmacy into your consideration.
- Don't ignore the patient's psychology and to ask about the caregiver especially in elderly.

- Always remember management should be patient centered meaning that you should share the patient with every single step in your plan of management.
- Don't forget to alert the patient about the red flags.

*Abbreviation Elaboration

*RBS: Random Blood Sugar

References

1. National Clinical Guidelines for non-surgical treatment of patients with recent onset low back pain or lumbar radiculopathy. Stochkendahl MJ, Kjaer P, Hartvigsen J, et al. Eur Spine J 2018; 27: 60-75.
2. American Academy of Family Physician (AAFP).
3. Low back pain and radicular pain: assessment and management. KCE report 287Cs. Brussels: Belgian Health Care Knowledge Centre (KCE),Van Wambeke P, Desomer A, Ailliet L, et al. Summary: 2017.
4. Noninvasive treatments for acute, subacute, and chronic low back pain: a clinical practice guideline from the American College of Physicians. Qaseem A, Wilt TJ, McLean RM, et al. Ann Intern Med 2017; 166: 514-530. 2017.

Case Study 5

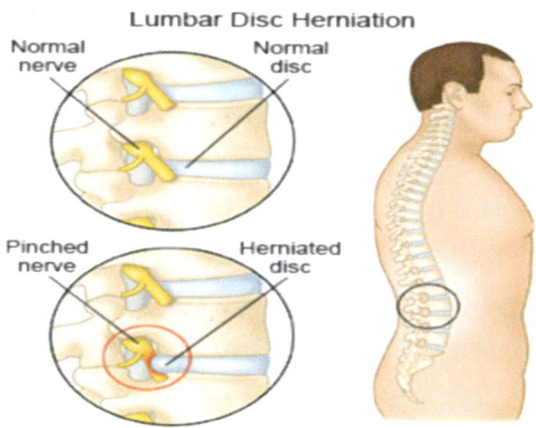

A 30-year-old male, sales representative in a pharmaceutical company, married, came to Family Medicine Clinic, complaining of acute severe low back pain.

Physician: When did your pain start?
Patient: one day ago.

Physician: Did you have any history of trauma?
Patient: Yes, Doctor. I felt a click sound when I tried to carry a box of medicine yesterday.

Physician: Okay, Mr. Murad. Let me check your back.
Physician palpates his back and feels stiffness of the Paraspinal muscles.

Physician: Okay, Mr. Murad. I think you have back muscle strain. I will prescribe painkillers for you, and advice you to rest and avoid movement, I will give you a sick leave for 1 week.
Mistakes:

- The physician did not introduce himself to the patient.
- Did not establish a good rapport with the patient.
- Did not ask detailed history about the pain, site, duration, character of pain, severity in scale from 1-10, aggravating and relieving factors, radiation of pain and associated symptoms.
- Did not ask the patient about the nature of his work.
- Early judgment of the cause of pain and the diagnosis
- Did not ask about the patient's ICE (idea, concern and expectation).
- Did not do proper clinical examination for the patient.
- Did not share the patient in the plan of management.
- Did not discharge the patient with safety netting advices.

Ideal Scenario

A 30 years old male, sales representative in a pharmaceutical company, married, came to Family Medicine Clinic, complaining of acute sever low back pain.

Physician: Welcome, Mr. Murad! My name is Dr. Mona, how can I help you?
Patient: How are you, Dr. Mona? I have low back pain.

Physician: For how long, Mr. Murad?
Patient: For almost one day doctor.

Physician: Would you please tell me more about this pain?
Patient: I had low back pain for two years that increased one day ago and I cannot lie flat, or sit as usual because of the pain.

Physician: What does the pain looks like?
Patient: It is shooting aches as an electrical pain.

Physician: Are there anything that increases or decreases this pain?
Patient: Usually the pain increases on bending forward, coughing or sneezing, and lying flat. The pain increases at early morning. I could not sleep at night Doctor. I noticed the pain decreases on walking.

Physician: Are there any associated symptoms?
Patient: Yes, doctor. I feel numbness and weakness of my left leg, I could not bend forward to tie my shoes this morning.

Physician: Can you tell me more about the nature of your work?
Patient: I am working as a sales representative in a pharmaceutical company, I got used to lifting heavy boxes every day to deliver them to the customers.

Physician: Did you have any history of trauma?
Patient: I think I injured my back yesterday when I tried to lift one of the medicine boxes.

Physician: Did you try any painkillers?
Patient: Yes, I tried Voltaren injection yesterday that decreases the pain slightly for sometimes, and then the pain comes back.

Physician: On a scale from 1 to 10, can you rate the severity of pain?
Patient: In most of the time it is 8 out of 10.

Physician: Does the pain go down to your legs?
Patient: Yes, it goes down my buttock and down my thigh till below the knee.

Physician: Do you feel any tingling sensation or numbness of your legs?
Patient: Yes.

Physician: Are you controlling your bowel Mr. Murad?
Patient: Yes.

Physician: Do you feel any increase in your body temperature?
Patient: No.
Physician: Do you have any history of chronic illnesses?
Patient: No.

Physician: Did you undergo any previous surgeries before?
Patient: No.

Physician: Do you have any family history of the same condition?
Patient: No.

Physician: What about your mood and interest in life?
Patient: I am fine doctor, enjoying life with my family.

Physician: Are you doing any sort of exercise?
Patient: Sometimes I am going to the gym.

Physician: Are you a smoker?
Patient: Yes, I smoke one pack per day for almost 10 years.

Physician: Do you have any history of weight loss?
Patient: No.

Physician: Any history of recent travel?
Patient: No.

Physician: Okay, Mr. Murad let me summarize your condition. You are 30 years old, sales representative, smoker for almost 10 years and you had low back pain for two years that increased one day ago with history of lifting a heavy object yesterday, pain increases at the morning, disturbing your sleep, also increase with sitting, bending forward, coughing or sneezing and lying flat, no associated fever, no weight loss, no loss of bowel control.

Physician: Do you want to add anything else?
Patient: No

Physician: Do you have any idea or concern about the cause of your back pain?
Patient: I am afraid doctor that I might have disc prolapse.

Physician: What do you expect from me?
Patient: I need something to relieve my pain.

Physician: Okay, Mr. Murad. Can I examine you please?

On Examination:

- Patient is vitally stable: temperature: 36.5 °C, pulse 90 beats per minute, regular, BP=138/80. Oxygen sat 100%, weight 100 kg, height 170 cm, BMI=34.6, pain scale 8/10, smoker
- Gait is abnormal, patient extending his back because of the pain

Back Examination:

- Inspection: Patient is sitting on the edge of the chair, overstretching his back in pain
- Palpation: Both shoulders are asymmetrical, tilting of the right hip, tenderness of paraspinal muscle at lumber area left side with stiffness.
- Mobility: Limited with tenderness elicited on flexion, extension and rotation of the back.
- Special tests: Positive straight leg raising (SST) and femoral stretch test (FST)
- Muscle power of the lower extremities: 4/5
- Neuro-vascular examination: Sensation and pulsation of the lower limb are preserved

Discussion and Counselling:

Physician: Okay, Mr. Murad. After taking your history and examining you, I think that you may have a disc disorder that gets worse after you lift the heavy box.

Also you have increase in weight, you have obesity together with smoking that needs another medical care.

Patient: So what can you offer me doctor, I tried to lose weight myself many times, I also tried to quit smoking, but I failed.

Physician: Okay, Mr. Murad, let us discuss your problems one by one.
First regarding your disc prolapse:
We need to do plain X-ray now, Mr. Murad.
The physician checks the X-ray and notice narrowing of the disc space between L5, S1.

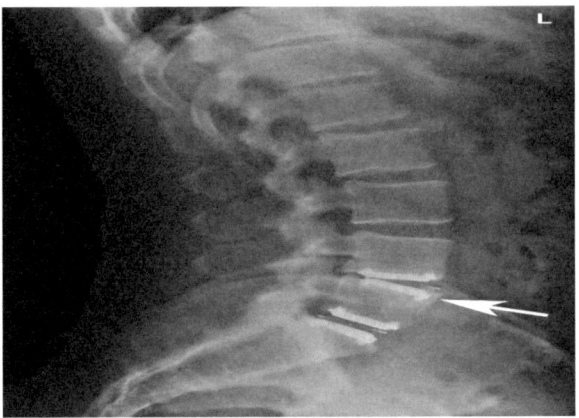

Figure 4: Lateral Lumbosacral x ray showing Narrowing of The L5-S1disc space (Arrow)

The physician explained the result of the X-ray and expressed his concern about the symptoms that the patient suffered from and the detected signs and the need for MRI lumbosacral area to roll out disc herniation, patient accepted to do MRI.

After doing MRI the physician discovered a small herniated disc prolapse between L5-S1 and started discussing the plan of management.

Physician: Okay Mr. Murad, let me explain our plan of management for your condition:

The first step to recovery includes non-surgical treatment such as non-steroidal anti-inflammatory and muscle relaxants.

- About 80% of people suffering from lumbar disc prolapse experience a reduction in their symptoms within four to six weeks and return to normal activities. If pain persists, we can refer you to physiotherapy that can help to strengthen your lower back, leg and stomach muscles and increase the flexibility of the spine.
- In case of loss of sensation in the legs, we can refer you to spinal surgery as a surgical treatment called discectomy may have to be performed. The part of the ruptured disc causing pain is carefully removed and 80-85% of the patients are able to recover and resume their normal activity in about six weeks.

- Ensure good posture while sitting, sleeping and walking. Use the right technique during lifting any heavy weight and always maintain a healthy weight.

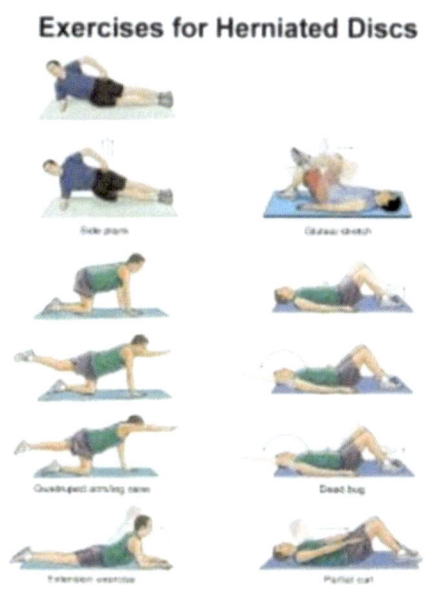

Figure 5: Herniated Disc Exercises

Second: We should pay attention to your weight and smoking, so our hospital can offer you extra care through life style modification clinic and smoking cessation clinic that will help you in these two issues.

We will reassess you after 6 weeks. If you are not improving, or if you find your pain is worsening, feel weakness of your limb, uncontrolling your bowel or difficult movement, please come back at any time. We can refer you to spinal surgery.

Also I advise you to keep going: This may not be possible at first if the pain is very bad. However, move around as soon as possible and get back into normal activities as soon as you are able. As a rule, don't do anything that causes a lot of pain. However, you will have to accept some discomfort when you are trying to keep active, but this is not harmful. Setting a new goal each day may be a good idea – for example, walking around the house one day, a walk to the shops the next, etc.

Physician: Do you want to ask me any questions Mr. Murad?
Patient: Thank you, Dr. Mona

Clinical Pearls and Take-Home Messages

Approximately 80 to 90% of disc prolapses tend to resolve spontaneously, and symptoms typically diminish on their own. This natural resolution process generally spans 6-8 weeks, though it may extend.

In cases of acute disc prolapse, conservative treatment is the primary approach unless there is significant spinal cord or nerve root compression or impaired function. Initial conservative measures involve a combination of anti-inflammatory and paracetamol-based medications, mild opioids, and neuropathic medications like amitriptyline. This is complemented by a physiotherapy program, and in some instances, hydrotherapy and Pilates.

If symptoms persist despite conservative treatment, intervention may be recommended. Options include a nerve sheath injection with local anesthetic (as steroids have not shown additional benefit) or surgery. Surgery has demonstrated efficacy in expediting recovery following disc prolapse.

The choice of treatment for each individual is customized based on their clinical presentation, radiological findings, and specific circumstances.

Differential Diagnosis of Mechanical Low Back Pain

Diagnosis (percentage of patients with low back pain)	Key characteristics and clinical clues
Lumbosacral muscle strains/sprains (70%)	Often following isolated traumatic incidents or repetitive overuse; pain worse with movement, relieved by rest; examination may reveal restricted range of motion, muscle tenderness, or trigger points
Lumbar spondylosis (10%)	More common in persons older than 40 years; pain may be present in or radiate from the hips; pain is worse with activity; pain may worsen with lumbar spine extension or rotation; neurologic examination is usually normal
Disk herniation (5% to 10%)	Most often involves the L5 or S1 nerve root, at L4-L5 or L5-S1 in 90% to 95% of cases; symptoms may include pain, paresthesia, sensory change, loss of strength or reflexes depending on affected nerve root
Spondylolysis (less than 5%*)	Common in young athletes; symptoms often develop insidiously; pain with activities involving lumbar extension; imaging is diagnostic, but early imaging in the absence of red flags is typically not necessary; usually occurs in a lower lumbar vertebra, most often L5
Vertebral compression fracture (4%)	Fracture may occur slowly over time or acutely with mild trauma; acute episodes usually resolve in four to six weeks, but abnormal healing or additional fractures may result in chronic pain and functional impairment; presents as localized back pain that is worse with flexion and often point tenderness on palpation; risk factors include increased age, history of trauma, chronic steroid use, and osteoporosis; plain radiography should be obtained to confirm diagnosis
Spondylolisthesis (3% to 4%)	Pain often radiates into the buttocks or posterior thigh; leg pain may be worse than back pain; often presents as paresthesias, numbness, or weakness; occurs at L5 in 90% of cases
Spinal stenosis (3%)	Presents as back pain, sometimes with sensory loss or numbness in the legs; calf pain with ambulation that is relieved with rest/sitting (pseudoclaudication); neurologic examination findings are normal; imaging is diagnostic

*—Occurs in less than 5% of the general population but in up to 50% of preadolescent and adolescent athletes.

Information from references 1 through 3, 5 through 7, and 11.

Table 6: Differential diagnosis of lumbo-sacral disc prolapses
**American Academy of Family Physician (AAFP)
Home Message to Family Physician

1. Begin the interaction by introducing yourself to the patient.
2. Demonstrate empathy and work towards establishing a positive rapport with the patient.
3. Conduct a comprehensive and detailed patient history.
4. Utilize open-ended questions to encourage thorough communication.
5. Maintain a non-judgmental approach throughout the interaction.
6. Allow the patient to express their ideas, concerns, and expectations freely.
7. Ensure a focused examination is not overlooked.
8. Consider the patient holistically, taking into account daily habits and lifestyle, particularly in younger patients.
9. Acknowledge and address the patient's psychological aspects.
10. Emphasize patient-centered management, involving the patient in every step of the treatment plan.
11. Highlight red flags and alert the patient to potential warning signs.
12. Recognize that a significant portion of back pain results from overuse or misuse.
13. Inquire about the patient's social life, as it may provide valuable insights into their condition.
14. Consider risk factors such as gender, sedentary lifestyle, weight, physical strain, and smoking in assessing the likelihood of lumbar disc prolapse.
15. Approximately 50 out of 100 individuals experience improvement within 10 days, and 75 out of 100 after four weeks. Only around 2 out of 100 people with a prolapsed disc still experience severe pain after 12 weeks, necessitating surgery.

References

1. National Clinical Guidelines for non-surgical treatment of patients with recent onset low back pain or lumbar radiculopathy. Stochkendahl MJ, Kjaer P, Hartvigsen J, et al. Eur Spine J 2018; 27: 60-75.
2. American Academy of Family Physician (AAFP).
3. Low back pain and radicular pain: assessment and management. KCE report 287Cs. Brussels: Belgian Health Care Knowledge Centre (KCE),Van Wambeke P, Desomer A, Ailliet L, et al. Summary: 2017.
4. Noninvasive treatments for acute, su
5. bacute, and chronic low back pain: a clinical practice guideline from the American College of Physicians. Qaseem A, Wilt TJ, McLean RM, et al. Ann Intern Med 2017; 166: 514-530. 2017.
6. National Institute for Health and Care Excellence (NICE). Low back pain and sciatica in over 16s: assessment and management. NICE guideline [NG59]. London: NICE, 2016.

Neurological Presentations

Suwaidi M. Alghanmi, MD

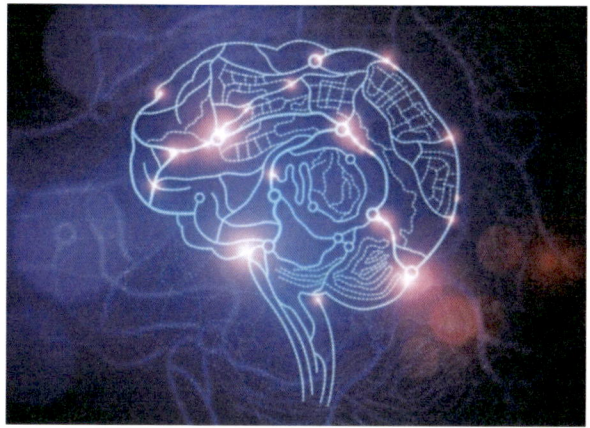

Case Study 1

A 37-year-old female presented in the afternoon with fascial weakness.

Physician: Since when have you had this weakness?
Patient: Since morning when I woke up.

Physician: Who noticed this weakness?
Patient: I noticed it when I washed my face and was confirmed by my husband.

Physician: Have you had the same illness in your family before?
Patient: No, my husband said his sister had fascial weakness.

Physician: Do you have any chronic diseases?
Patient: Diabetes but controlled on diet and exercise.

Physician: Did you do any dental procedures before this symptom?
Patient: No.

Physician: Doctor, what is your treatment?
Patient: Prednisolone and physiotherapy

What is the proper Diagnosis?

A. Bell's palsy
B. Lyme disease
C. Gullian barre syndrome
D. none of the above

Availability Heuristics (bias)

In the above case, the physician thought about a diagnosis that he knows, so most questions guided his impression even without full cranial and neurological examination.

Ideal Scenario

A 37-year-old female presented in the afternoon with fascial weakness.
Physician: Since when have you had this weakness?
Patient: Since morning when I woke up.
Physician: Can you elaborate more about your symptoms?
Patient: I woke up this morning with numbness in my face around the angle of my mouth, left mouth deviation and difficulty swallowing also short of breath on Exertion, my sister in law had fascial weakness but she didn't have difficulty swallowing or numbness but she lost taste in part of her tongue and she was hearing the sound loudly and I don't have these symptoms also she was treated by prednisolone and physiotherapy.

What were the mistakes in the first scenario?

A. physician used leading questions
B. physician didn't let the patient to elaborate her concerns
C. physician was biased by the diagnosis of the sister-in-law
D. All of the above

How to prevent falling in the availability bias?

A. Encourage the patient to reveal her concerns.
B. Spend more time exploring the symptoms.
C. Make your primary concern to help the patient.

A 37 years old female with fascial weakness, numbness around angle of mouth, difficulty swallowing and short of breath with exertion.

What is the appropriate diagnosis?

A. vascular insult
B. demyelinating disease
C. bulbar myasthenia gravis
D. none of the above

Case Study 2

A 37-year-old female with fascial weakness, numbness around angle of mouth, difficulty swallowing and short of breath with exertion.

Physician: Since when these symptoms?
Patient: For five days.

Physician: Have you sought medical advice?
Patient: Yes.

Physician: Have you used any medications or did any investigations?
Patient: I used prednisolone and MRI was done.

Physician: What is the result?
Patient: MRI showed a vascular loop around the 7th cranial nerve.

What was the potential mistakes in the first scenario?

- The physician needs to differentiate between fascial weakness of upper motor neuron type and lower motor neuron type so he needs full neurological examination and to find diagnosis that explains all the patient's symptoms, he also should ask about the benefit of medications.
- Physician was biased by MRI result which did not explain the patient's symptoms so the ideal scenario is to refer the patient to a Neurologist for further investigation and management.

Take Home Message

Myasthenia Gravis (MG) is the most common disorder of neuromuscular transmission and one of the best defined autoimmune diseases. The characteristic sign of the disorder is a fluctuating weakness in the ocular, bulbar, limb, and respiratory muscles.

Signs and symptoms of progressive bulbar palsy include difficulty swallowing, weak jaw and facial muscles, progressive loss of speech, and weakening of the tongue.

Case Study 3

45-year-old male complaining of eyelid drop seen in neurology clinic today with history of increased urination in the Family Medicine Clinic.

Physician: Since when did you notice this symptom?
Patient: A Couple of months.

Physician: Have you seen a urologist?
Patient: No.

Physician: Have you complained of dysuria?
Patient: No.

Physician: Did you check your RFT* recently?
Patient: Yes, and it was normal.

Physician: Did you complain of thirst or weight loss?
Patient: No.

What is the most likely cause of this patient's symptoms?

A. ocular myasthenia
B. UTI
C. medication side effect
D. BPH*
E. none of the above

Ideal Scenario

40-years-old male complaining of eyelid drop seen in neurology clinic today with history of increased urination in the Family Medicine Clinic.

Physician: Since when did you noticed this symptom?
Patient: A couple of months.

Physician: Can you elaborate more about your symptoms?
Patient: I think it started after I used a medication from a Neurology clinic.

Physician: Why have you been following a neurologist?
Patient: Because of the eyelid drop, initially I was seen by an ophthalmologist and he referred me to a neurologist who diagnosed me as having ocular myasthenia.

Physician: Which medications have you used currently?
Patient: Mestinon.

Physician: Are you worried about any diseases?
Patient: Diabetes.

What were the biased mistakes in the first scenario?

A. The physician thought about a diagnosis that he knows (Diabetes and its complication).
B. Avoid directing questions.
C. Physician isn't familiar with the side effects of myasthenia gravis medications.
D. All of the above.

Case Study 4

A 41-year-old female free medically complains of fatigability, shortness of breath on exertions and inability to comb her Hair. These symptoms worsen at the end of the day.

What is the most likely cause of this patient's symptoms?

A. polymyositis
B. dermatomyositis
C. myasthenia gravis
D. congestive heart failure
E. muscular Dystrophy

Physical examination showed weak neck flexion, double vision, eyelid drop, difficulty to count till number 20 and difficulty to abduct her shoulder in purpose to comb her hair, other neurological examinations are unremarkable.

What is the most likely cause of this patient's symptoms?

A. polymyositis
B. dermatomyositis
C. myasthenia gravis
D. congestive heart failure
E. muscular dystrophy

Her labs showed positive acetylcholine receptor antibodies, anti-musk is negative.

What investigation you still need and will affect your management?

A. CBC
B. urine analysis

C. EEG
D. CT chest
E. Echocardiogram

Answers:

Given this scenario you have to think in myasthenia gravis as a diagnosis especially in female gender with positive fatigability Test and send for acetylcholine receptor antibody, anti-musk and single fiber to confirm your Diagnosis and ask for a CT chest for thymoma if present, its removal will reduce the relapse of symptoms. Absence of antibodies will not exclude the Diagnosis of MG especially with highly suspicious symptoms.

Myasthenia gravis Symptoms

- The initial symptom is typically specific muscle weakness and fatigability rather than generalized weakness
- Weakness worsens with exercise and as the day progresses
- Generally, weakness often affects the eye muscles to facial muscles and then limb muscles.
- Eye problems such as drooping and double vision.
- Problems with speaking, swallowing (leading to choking easily), and chewing.

Common Tests & Procedures:

Edrophonium (Tensilon) test: A drug called Tensilon (or a placebo) is administered intravenously, through a vein, and the muscle movements are observed.

Repetitive nerve stimulation test: Small pulses of electricity used to check the nerve ability to pass stimuli to muscle.

Antibody test: Blood test to check for antibodies associated with MG.

CT scan: To rule out the presence of a tumor in the thymus.

Magnetic resonance imaging (MRI): MRI of the chest is performed to rule out a presence of tumor in the thymus.

Pulmonary function tests (PFTs): To check any breathing difficulty.

Medication

- **Immunosuppressant**: Abnormal immune response can be minimized.
- **Cholinesterase inhibitors**: Helps improving signaling between cells.

Procedures

- Thymectomy: Enlarged thymus may be removed to relieve the symptoms.
- Plasma exchange: Removal of antibodies from plasma, to reduce the excess of antibodies.

Nutrition

Foods to Eat:

- Myasthenia gravis can weaken lips, tongue, and jaw. To reduce fatigue from chewing it may be helpful to moisten solid foods with gravy, sauce, broth, butter, mayonnaise, sour cream or yogurt.
- Choose chicken or fish instead of tougher meats.

Foods to Avoid:

- Avoid dry crumbly food such as crackers, hard rice, cookies, nuts, chips or popcorn.
- Avoid bread products such as sandwiches, bagels and muffins.

Clinical Pearls and Take-Home Messages

Myasthenia gravis is not a preventable disease, but avoiding the following triggers can prevent patients from exacerbation.

- Emotional stress
- Exposure to extreme temperatures
- Fever

- Infections (e.g., respiratory infection, pneumonia, tooth abscess)
- Medications (e.g., muscle relaxants, anticonvulsants, certain antibiotics)

*Abbreviation Elaboration
*RFT: Renal Function Test
*BPH: Benign Prostatic Hyperplasia

References

1. Drachman DB. Myasthenia gravis. N Engl J Med. 1994;330:1797 810. [PubMed] [Google Scholar].
2. Keesey JC. Clinical evaluation and management of myasthenia gravis. Muscle Nerve. 2004; 29:484–505. [PubMed] [Google Scholar].
3. Grob D, Brunner N, Namba T, Pagala M. Lifetime course of myasthenia gravis. Muscle Nerve. 2008; 37:141–9. [PubMed] [Google Scholar].

Arthralgia Chapter

Ghada A. Rayes, MD
Tariq A. Albeshri, MD

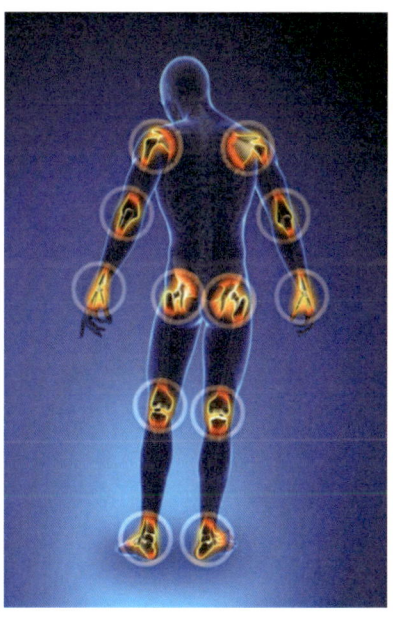

Case Study 1

Mrs. Alwa is a 40-year-old lady, known case of Hypothyroidism on L-Thyroxin 50mcg OD, Rheumatoid Arthritis diagnosed 3 years ago, on prednisolone 5 mg od / MTX* 15mg once weekly / Adalimumab 40 mg EOW* maintenance dose as the patient is in state of remission since 1year. Treated Vitamin D3 Deficiency.

Presented to the primary care physician with a history of left knee pain and swelling in the past two days.

Physician: Any history of trauma?
Patient: Nothing that I recall.

Physician: Does the pain interfere with your daily activity?
Patient: Yes, it interferes even with walking and climbing.

Physician: Is there any redness or hotness?
Patient: Yes, beside the swollen knee it is slightly red and warm.

Physician: Do you have a fever?
Patient: I feel hot but I took Naproxen 500mg twice daily, so that it makes me feel better.

Physician: Are you taking your DMARD* medications regularly?
Patient: Yes.

The Physician started to examine Mrs. Alwa.

- O/E:
- Vitally normal, Temp=37.4, BMI=21
- General: looks in pain

- Left knee: swollen, red, with a tiny pustule. Tenderness all over the joint, and limited range of motion (fixed flexion position).
- Hands Examination: unremarkable for swelling, erythema or deformity, no signs of effusion, intact range of motion, no focal tenderness
- Shoulder Examination: Unremarkable for joint inflammation.

The physician ordered an x-ray of the left knee, and labs including CBC-deferential, ESR, CRP, Vit-D3.

- Renewed appointment with rheumatology to be after 3 days. He continued the patient on NSAID until her appointment.

What went wrong in the previous scenario?
The physician did not pay attention to the history of fever that was masked with the regular use of NSAIDs.

The physician asked the right questions, did the appropriate examination, yet the plan decided for the patient was not appropriate. The lab works that was requested were relatively appropriate except for Vitamin D3 level as the patient was treated and unlikely Vit. D3 deficiency would cause her symptoms. Lab works were ordered as routine instead of urgent.

Initial impression and plan:

- The case was acute mono-arthritis + fever so urgent workup and Joint aspiration was indicated. Urgent Orthopedic was needed to rule out septic arthritis.
- In the previous scenario the physician obviously assumed that the patient had a flare of Rheumatoid arthritis for which an appointment with her rheumatologist was arranged in 3 days.

Ideal Scenario

Physician: Any history of trauma?
Patient: Nothing that I recall.

Physician: Does the pain interfere with your daily activity?

Patient: Yes, it interferes even with walking and climbing.

Physician: Is there any redness or hotness?
Patient: Yes, beside of swollen knee it is slightly red and warm.

Physician: Any skin lesions?
Patient: A small pimple over my knee that oozes sometimes noticed around five days ago.

Physician: Do you have fever?
Patient: I feel hot, but I take Naproxen 500mg twice daily so that it makes me feel better.

Physician: Are you taking your DMARD medications regularly?
Patient: Yes, I am taking prednisolone 5 mg od / MTX 15 once weekly / adalimumab 40 mg EOW.

Physician: Are there any other joint involvement or stiffness?
Patient: Not at all.

The Physician started to examine Mrs. Alwa.
O/E:
Vitally normal, Temp=37.4 (NSAID was taken 2 hours prior to examination), BMI=21.
General: looks in pain.
Left knee: swollen, red, inflamed with a tiny pustule. Tenderness all over the joint, and limited range of motion. (Fixed flexion position).
Hands Examination: unremarkable for swelling, erythema or deformity, no signs of effusion, intact range of motion, no focal tenderness.
Shoulder Examination: Unremarkable for joint inflammation.
The physician ordered *urgent* X-ray left knee, and urgent labs including CBC-deferential, ESR, CRP.
Laboratory Exam:
Hb=11.6
WBCs=14000, MCV, MCH=n, RDW=11.3 low, Plt=206 n
ESR=50++

CRP=70

Urine analysis= Unremarkable

UAC*=0.819 n

Serum Creatinine=55 e-GFR*=100

X-ray left knee: soft tissue swelling around the joint and a widened joint space.

The Physician contacted Orthopedic on-call and referred the patient to him for urgent left knee *joint aspiration* to rule out septic arthritis.

Renewed appointment with rheumatology to be after 3 days.

*Abbreviation Elaboration

* MTX: Methotrexate
* EOW: Every Other Week
* DMARD: Disease Modifying Anti-Rheumatoid Drugs
* UAC: Urinary Albumin Creatinine Ratio
* e-GFR: Estimated Glomerular filtration Rate

References

1. Chouk, M., Verhoeven, F., Sondag, M., Guillot, X., Prati, C. and Wendling, D. (2019). Value of serum procalcitonin for the diagnosis of bacterial septic arthritis in daily practice in rheumatology. Clinical Rheumatology, 38(8), pp.2265–2273.
2. Ross, J.J. (2017). Septic Arthritis of Native Joints. Infectious Disease Clinics of North America, 31(2), pp.203–218.

Case Study 2

A 32-year-old lady, not known to have any medical illnesses seeking your advice regarding abnormal lab results (done in another institute). ANA 1:160.

Physician: Any history of rash?
Patient: Nothing that I recall.

Physician: Any history of joint pain?
Patient: Well, I feel aches and pain all over my body.

Physician: Do you experience any change in the color of your fingers when exposed to cold or stress?
Patient: Sometimes my fingertips turn to blue color with no pain or numbness.

Physician: Any family history of rheumatic diseases?
Patient: My mother has rheumatoid arthritis.

The Physician started to examine her. *O/E:* Vitally normal, Temp=37, BMI= 29.
General: looks well but depressed Musculoskeletal Examination: unremarkable for swelling, erythema or deformities, no signs of effusion, intact range of motion, no focal tenderness Multiple soft tissue tenderness.
The physician ordered: CBC-deferential, ESR, CRP, Vit-D3 ANA / DNA / ANTI-SMITH / SSA / SSB / Complement level X-ray hand / elbow / shoulder / knee / feet. Referred to rheumatology clinic for further evaluation.
What went wrong in the previous scenario?

- The physician was biased by the lab result.

- The physician used leading questions based on lab results.
- The physician did not give the patient time to explain her main issue and why did her primary physician order ANA.
- Physician did not ask about other causes of high ANA.

Ideal Scenario

Physician: What is your complaint?
Patient: I feel fatigue, not feeling well and I noticed my weight increased.

Physician: Since when did it start?
Patient: Around one year.

Physician: What are other complaints?
Patient: I feel cold all the time and this was noticed also by my family.

Also, I noticed a change in my voice and disturbance in my menstrual cycle.

Physician: Any history of thyroid disease in the family?
Patient: Yes, my mother and sister have hypothyroidism.

Physician: Do you have joint pain, swelling, or stiffness?
Patient: Not at all.

Physician: Do you have skin rash, oral ulcer…(Symptoms suggesting underlying CTDs)?
Patient: Not at all.

Physician: Are you taking any medications?
Patient: No.

The Physician started to examine her. *O/E:* Vitally normal, Temp=37, BMI=29 General: looks well not in pain or distress but depressed with dry skin and loss of eye brows hair.

Musculoskeletal (MSK) Examination: unremarkable for swelling, erythema or deformities, no signs of effusion, intact range of motion, no focal tenderness.

Multiple soft tissue tenderness.

Thyroid exam: unremarkable/no masses or lymphadenopathies. *The physician referred the patient to endocrinology for further assessment labs were ordered including thyroid function test.*

Clinical Pearls and Take-Home Messages

1. Systemic lupus erythematosus (SLE) is a systemic autoimmune disease, with multisystem involvement. The disease has several phenotypes, with varying clinical presentations in patients ranging from mild mucocutaneous manifestations to multi-organ and severe central nervous system involvement.
2. Diagnosis of SLE can be challenging and based on the constellation of signs, symptoms and appropriate laboratory workup (no single clinical feature or lab abnormality can confirm a diagnosis of SLE).
3. ANA, although sensitive, is far from specific for SLE. A positive ANA is also seen in many other illnesses including systemic sclerosis and polymyositis, as well as some chronic infections (a positive ANA does not confirm the diagnosis of SLE, but a negative ANA makes it very less likely).

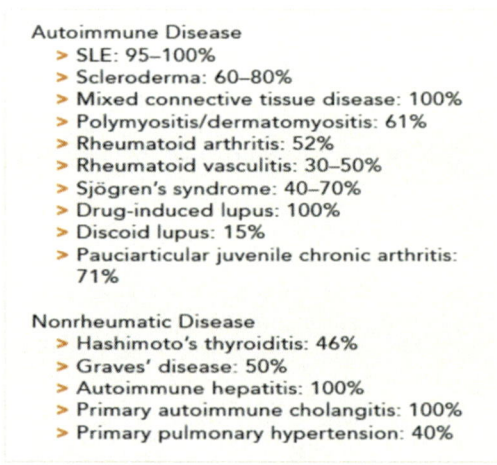

Table 7: Sensitivity of the ANA in autoimmune and Nonrheumatic disease

Entry criterion
Antinuclear antibodies (ANA) at a titer of ≥1:80 on HEp-2 cells or an equivalent positive test (ever)

If absent, do not classify as SLE
If present, apply additive criteria

Additive criteria
Do not count a criterion if there is a more likely explanation than SLE.
Occurrence of a criterion on at least one occasion is sufficient.
SLE classification requires at least one clinical criterion and ≥10 points.
Criteria need not occur simultaneously.
Within each domain, only the highest weighted criterion is counted toward the total score§.

Clinical domains and criteria	Weight	Immunology domains and criteria	Weight
Constitutional		**Antiphospholipid antibodies**	
Fever	2	Anti-cardiolipin antibodies OR	
Hematologic		Anti-β2GP1 antibodies OR	
Leukopenia	3	Lupus anticoagulant	2
Thrombocytopenia	4	**Complement proteins**	
Autoimmune hemolysis	4	Low C3 OR low C4	3
Neuropsychiatric		Low C3 AND low C4	4
Delirium	2	**SLE-specific antibodies**	
Psychosis	3	Anti-dsDNA antibody* OR	
Seizure	5	Anti-Smith antibody	6
Mucocutaneous			
Non-scarring alopecia	2		
Oral ulcers	2		
Subacute cutaneous OR discoid lupus	4		
Acute cutaneous lupus	6		
Serosal			
Pleural or pericardial effusion	5		
Acute pericarditis	6		
Musculoskeletal			
Joint involvement	6		
Renal			
Proteinuria >0.5g/24h	4		
Renal biopsy Class II or V lupus nephritis	8		
Renal biopsy Class III or IV lupus nephritis	10		

Total score:

Classify as Systemic Lupus Erythematosus with a score of 10 or more if entry criterion fulfilled.

Figure 6: ACR/EULAR classification criteria for SLE

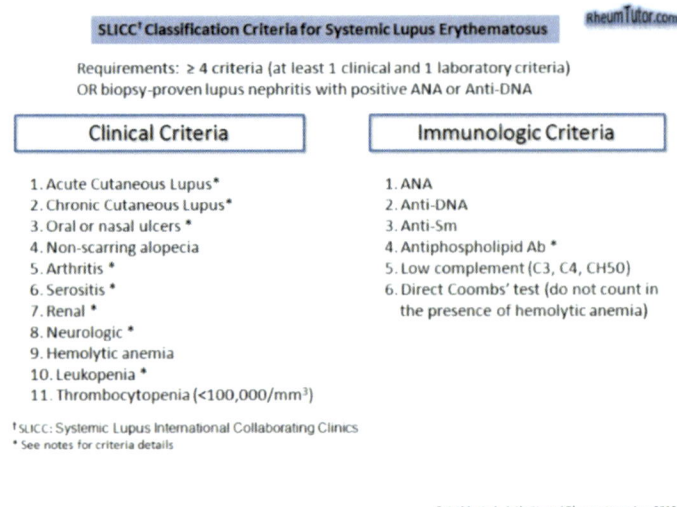

Figure 7: SUCC classification criteria of SLE

References

1. Aringer, M., Costenbader, K., Daikh, D., Brinks, R., Mosca, M., Ramsey-Goldman, R., Smolen, J.S., Wofsy, D., Boumpas, D.T., Kamen, D.L., Jayne, D., Cervera, R., Costedoat-Chalumeau, N., Diamond, B., Gladman, D.D., Hahn, B., Hiepe, F., Jacobsen, S., Khanna, D. and Lerstrøm, K. (2019). 2019 European League against Rheumatism/American College of Rheumatology Classification Criteria for Systemic Lupus Erythematosus. Arthritis & Rheumatology, [online] 71(9), pp.1400–1412. Available at: https://www.rheumatology.org/Portals/0/Files/Classification-Criteria-Systemic-Lupus-Erythematosus.pdf.
2. Sliccgroup.org. (2012). SLE Criteria: SLICC. [online] Available at: https://sliccgroup.org/research/sle-criteria/.Grygiel-Górniak, B., Rogacka, N. and Puszczewicz, M. (2018). Antinuclear antibodies in healthy people and non-rheumatic diseases – diagnostic and clinical implications. Reumatologia/Rheumatology, 56(4), pp.243–248.

Case Study 3

Mrs. Nawal is a 32-year-old lady, P3, last pregnancy was 2 years ago, smoker, history of H-pylori infection for which she completed treatment 1 month ago.

Patient known to have IBD, diagnosed 10 years ago on treatment.

The patient presented to the primary care physician with a history of lower back pain for five years.

Physician: How did the pain start?
Patient: It started five years ago, I felt it while I was in bed, and I couldn't get up from bed immediately.

Physician: Does it radiate anywhere?
Patient: No, mainly I feel it over the lower back.

Physician: Was there any history of trauma?
Patient: No.

Physician: Does it interfere with daily activity?
Patient: Actually, I feel the pain every morning, sometimes it's hard for me to get up from bed and go to work.

Physician: Any aggravating or relieving factors?
Patient: The pain increases with prolonged sitting or lying down, relieved by activity, and I often need to take painkillers like Ibuprofen to relieve the pain although it hurts my stomach.

Physician: Any fever or weight loss?

Patient: I have no fever, but I have lost weight around 5 kg in 2 months as my GI symptoms, epigastric pain, nausea and diarrhea did not resolve completely even after I completed the course of H-pylori treatment.

The Physician started to examine Mrs. Manal.

On Examination:

Vital Signs Normal BMI=26

General: The patient doesn't look in pain, walks and sits easily, Gait is intact.

Back inspection: no obvious deformities Range of Motion (ROM): limitation in flexion (painful flexion), other ROM intact On palpation: tenderness over lumbosacral spine and both sacroiliac joints Rt>Lt The physician ordered labs including Complete Blood Count, Vitamin D3, Stool for H-Pylori X-ray Lumbosacral Spine to rule out Spondylolisthesis vs Spondylosis.

The Physician started treating the patient as back pain due to muscular spasm prescribed Celecoxib, topical NSAIDs, Muscle Relaxant, and Proton Pump Inhibitors for her epigastric pain.

What went wrong in the previous scenario?

- The physician took details of the lower back pain but did not ask about other musculoskeletal or joint involvement.
- The physician did not pay attention to extra articular symptoms like GI symptoms, it seems that he assumed that her symptoms were related to H-pylori relapse and did not ask about the use of NSAIDS as a cause of gastric ulcer, GI bleeding, mouth ulcers and perianal lesions as inflammatory bowel disease should be considered in the differential diagnosis.
- Family history of inflammatory disease like Ankylosing Spondylitis, Reactive Arthritis, or Inflammatory bowel disease was not addressed in the history.
- There was no examination for back stiffness (Ankylosing Spondylitis) like Schober test, and other detailed clinical examinations for sacroiliitis.
- In the work up that was ordered for the patient, there was Vit-D3 level which is not related to the patient's complaint as its deficiency would not cause this kind of presentation. ESR, CRP were not ordered although it might help in the diagnosis of inflammatory back pain. The ordered x-

ray was for the lumbosacral region to rule out Spondylolisthesis vs. Spondylosis, but sacroiliac joint was not included in the imaging to rule out Sacroiliitis.
- Physician started treating the patient as back pain due to muscular spasm although the clinical presentation was going more with inflammatory back pain and further evaluation and management by rheumatologist was more appropriate.

Ideal Scenario

The patient presented to the primary care physician with a history of lower back pain for five years.

Physician: How did the pain start?
Patient: It started *five years ago*, I felt it while I was in bed, and I couldn't get up from bed immediately.

Physician: Does it radiate anywhere?
Patient: No, mainly I feel it over the lower back.

Physician: Was there any history of trauma?
Patient: No.

Physician: Does it interfere with daily activities?
Patient: Actually, I feel the pain every morning, sometimes it's hard for me to get up from bed and go to work.

Physician: Any aggravating or relieving factors?
Patient: The pain increases with prolonged sitting or lying down, relieved by activity, and I often need to take painkillers like Ibuprofen to relieve the pain although it hurts my stomach. *(Inflammatory LBP)*.

Physician: Any other joint pain or swelling?
Patient: I have had pain lately over my heels when I get up in the morning but when I start walking and after activity it disappears spontaneously *(Picture of bilateral plantar fasciitis)*.

Physician: Any fever or weight loss?

Patient: I have no fever, but I have *weight lost around 5 Kg in 2 months* as my GI symptoms, epigastric pain, nausea and *diarrhea* did not resolve completely even after I completed the course of H-pylori treatment. *(Red flag to r/o Inflammatory Bowel Disease Relapse).*

Physician: When were you *diagnosed with IBD* and how were you treated?
Patient: I was diagnosed 10 years ago based on *chronic bloody diarrhea* then I was started on treatment with *on and off relapses.*

Physician: Any *family history* of similar presentation, inflammatory back pain *(Ankylosing Spondylitis, other Spondyloarthropathy)*, any family history *of inflammatory bowel disease?*

Patient: My *sister* has chronic back pain for which she is following with rheumatology and taking *immunosuppressant* treatment.

The Physician started to examine Mrs. Manal.

On Examination:

Vital Signs are Normal BMI=26
General: The patient doesn't look in pain, walks and sits easily, Gait is intact.
Back examination:
Inspection: loss of lumbar lordosis.
Range of Motion: limitation in flexion (painful flexion) and extension at lumbar area, other ROM intact (thoracic and cervical).
Palpation: tenderness over lumbosacral spine and both sacroiliac joints Rt>Lt
+ve Schober test: Lumbar flexion difference 3.5cm.

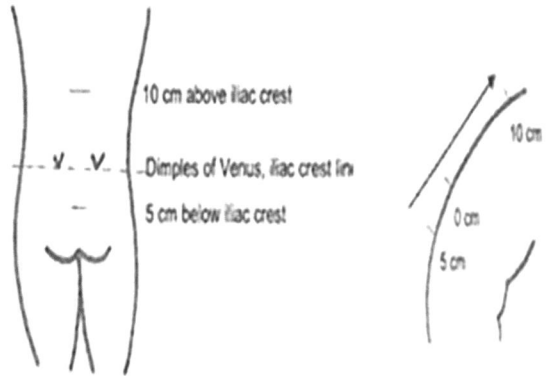

Figure 8: Schober test showing proper way of measurements

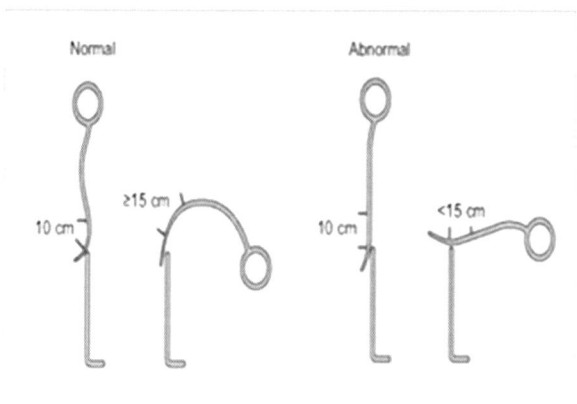

Figure 9: -ve Schober test in normal subject Vs +ve test

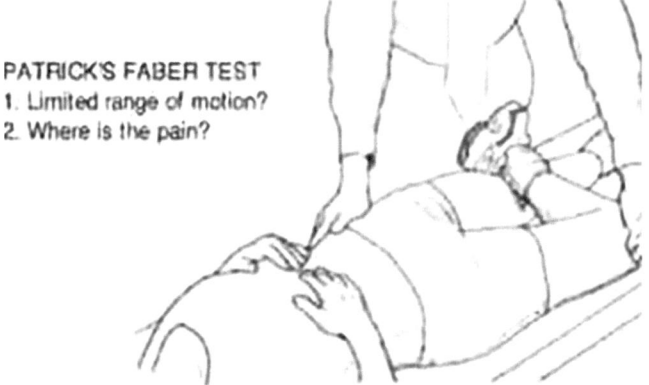

PATRICK'S FABER TEST
1. Limited range of motion?
2. Where is the pain?

1. Limited range of motion? Think hip arthritis, femoro acetabular impingement and other hip pathology.
2. Groin or side of hip pain, think hip conditions.
3. Lower back pain? Think sacroiliac conditions.

Figure 10: +ve FABER Test Rt side

Feet: unremarkable examination, the patient pointed at the site of pain over the plantar surface at the calcaneus *(Plantar Fasciitis)*.

The physician ordered labs including Complete Blood Count, *CRP*, *ESR*, Vitamin D3, and Stool for H-Pylori X-ray Lumbosacral Spine and Sacroiliac Joints.

Laboratory Exam:
Hb=12.5
WBCs=4000h, MCV, MCH=n, Plt=206 n
ESR=30++
CRP=25
VitD3=56
Stool H-Pylori=-ve

X-ray Thoracolumbar and Lumbosacral spine AP, Lateral View: = on Lateral view: small erosions at the corners of vertebral bodies surrounded by reactive sclerosis (Shiny Corners, Romanus Lesion).

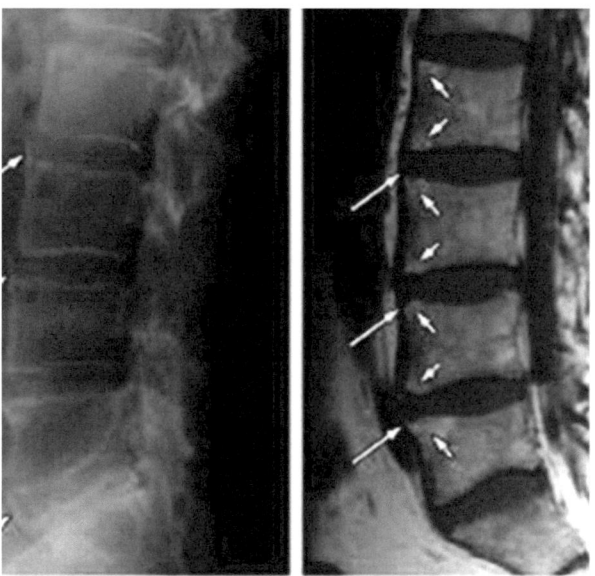

Figure 11: X-ray Thoracolumbar and Lumbosacral spine Lateral View showing small erosions at the corners of vertebral bodies (small arrows) surrounded by reactive sclerosis (Large arrows) – Shiny Corners, Romanus Lesion-.

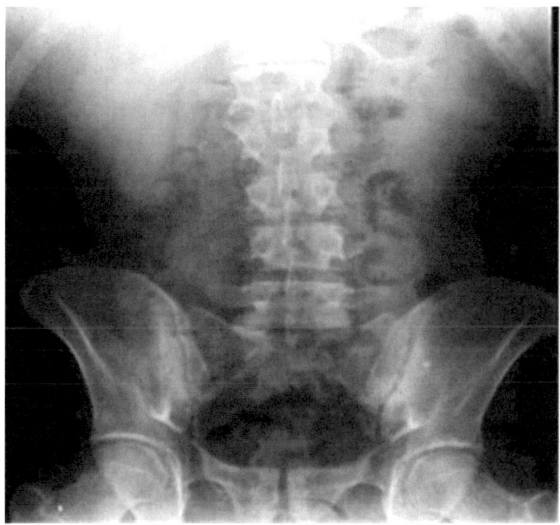

Figure 12: PA view of Sacroiliac Joints showing Bilateral Sacroiliac joints erosions, and iliac side subchondral sclerosis

The Physician referred the patient) to *Rheumatology* as a case of inflammatory back pain (? IBD related Sacroiliitis) for further assessment.

The Physician referred the patient to *Gastroenterology* for further assessment of persistent diarrhea (assessment of disease).

References

1. Themes, U.F.O. (2016). Back and lower extremity pain. [online] Anesthesia Key. Available at: https://aneskey.com/back-and-lower-extremity-pain/ [Accessed 12 Jan. 2022].
2. Ward, M.M., Deodhar, A., Gensler, L.S., Dubreuil, M., Yu, D., Khan, M.A., Haroon, N., Borenstein, D., Wang, R., Biehl, A., Fang, M.A., Louie, G., Majithia, V., Ng, B., Bigham, R., Pianin, M., Shah, A.A., Sullivan, N., Turgunbaev, M. and Oristaglio, J. (2019). 2019 Update of the American College of Rheumatology/Spondylitis Association of America/Spondyloarthritis Research and Treatment Network Recommendations for the Treatment of Ankylosing Spondylitis and Nonradiographic Axial Spondyloarthritis. Arthritis & Rheumatology, 71(10), pp.1599–1613.
3. Fragoulis, G.E., Liava, C., Daoussis, D., Akriviadis, E., Garyfallos, A. and Dimitroulas, T. (2019). Inflammatory bowel diseases and spondyloarthropathies: From pathogenesis to treatment. World Journal of Gastroenterology, 25(18), pp.2162–2176.
4. Review for the generalist: Evaluation of low back pain in children and adolescents – Scientific Figure on ResearchGate. Available from: https://www.researchgate.net/figure/Modified-Schobers-Test-Patient-standing-and-measurements-made-10-cm-above-and-5-cm_fig1_49623481.
5. Lewis, B. (n.d.). Faber test – Google Search. [online] www.google.com. Available at: https://www.google.com/search?q=faber+test&tbm=isch&ved=2ahUKEwjxkPbH0qz1AhWlkf0HHa9MC4EQ2-cCegQIABAA&oq [Accessed 12 Jan. 2022].
6. www.google.com. (n.d.). Shiny Corners – Google Search. [online] Available at: https://www.google.com/search?rlz=1C1GCEA_enSA970SA970&sxsr

f=AOaemvKukzus5q41pm8AIq-vW4cPilbzpw:1642162431349&source=univ&tbm=isch&q=Shiny+Corners [Accessed 14 Jan. 2022].

7. Pialat, J.-B., Di Marco, L., Feydy, A., Peyron, C., Porta, B., Himpens, P.-H., Ltaief-Boudrigua, A. and Aubry, S. (2016). Sacroiliac joints imaging in axial spondyloarthritis. Diagnostic and Interventional Imaging, [online] 97(7), pp.697–708. Available at: https://www.sciencedirect.com/science/article/pii/S2211568416000863 [Accessed 14 Jan. 2022].

Case Study 4

Mr. Ali is a 65 years old patient, known case of T2DM diagnosed 20 years ago, with Hypertension and peripheral neuropathy. The patient has poorly controlled blood glucose levels, he is on oral hypoglycemic medications (refusing insulin), antihypertensive treatment (ACE Inhibitors) and Gabapentin treatment for peripheral neuropathy. The patient came to his family medicine doctor complaining of bilateral hand joint stiffness for more than a year, progressively worsening, starting in both little fingers then involved almost all of his fingers. The patient stated that he is not improving on gabapentin.

Physician: Can you describe hand stiffness?
Patient: I find it difficult to open both of my hands (finger joints movement), numbness and tingling are always present (for which I'm taking treatment) even before the stiffness issue.

Physician: Any other joint involvement?
Patient: No, mainly I feel it over both of my hands.

Physician: Is there any history of fever, joint swelling or redness?
Patient: No.

Physician: Does it interfere with daily activities?
Patient: Not as much as I can wear my shirt, close the buttons etc. but it's hard for me to extend by hands so it affects handling the steering wheel while driving, also it's hard for me to extend my hands on the ground while praying.

Physician: Any aggravating or relieving factors?
Patient: No specific aggravating factors I feel it all the time, day and night.
The Physician started to examine Mr. Ali.

On Examination:

Vital Signs are Normal BMI=30.

Local: No swelling or redness, thickened waxy skin of both hands Range of Motion: limitation in extension of interphalangeal and proximal phalangeal joints of both hand Tests for carpal tunnel syndrome; Tinel test -ve, Phalen test -ve, Carpal compression test -ve.

The physician ordered labs including Complete Blood Count, ESR, CRP, RF, and Vitamin B12 X-ray hands EMG* nerve Conduction Study to rule out Carpal Tunnel Syndrome.

Initial impression and plan:

The physician had differential diagnosis; worsening peripheral neuropathy vs. bilateral Carpal Tunnel Syndrome, Rheumatoid arthritis. The physician doubled the dose of gabapentin to target neuropathy vs. Query Carpal Tunnel Syndrome and started NSAIDs for? Rheumatoid arthritis.

He gave the patient follow-up after 2 weeks for workup results.

What went wrong in the previous scenario?

- The physician missed asking about details of glycemic control and the reasons behind refusing insulin treatment, did not ask about other micro vascular complications like retinopathy that would be correlated with musculoskeletal diabetic hand deformities
- The physician did not observe the patient for hand deformities.

Ideal Scenario

The patient presented to his family physician with history of bilateral hand joints stiffness since more than a year.

Physician: Can you describe hand stiffness?

Patient: I find it difficult to open both of my hands (finger joints movement), numbness and tingling are always present (for which I'm taking treatment) even before the stiffness issue.

Physician: Any other joints involvement?

Patient: No, mainly I feel it over both of my hands

Physician: Is there any history of fever, joint swelling or redness?
Patient: No.
Physician: Does it interfere with daily activities?
Patient: Not as much as I can wear my shirt, close the buttons etc. but it's hard for me to extend by hands, so it affects handling the steering wheel while driving, also it's hard for me to extend my hands on the ground while praying.

Physician: Any aggravating or relieving factors?
Patient: No specific aggravating factors I feel it all the time, day and night.

Physician: How is your blood glucose control? Are you making home glucose monitoring?
Patient: No, my glucometer is not working, but usually my blood sugar around 200mg/dl (non-fasting).

Physician: You established micro vascular complications like peripheral neuropathy, any other complications related to your uncontrolled DM like Retinopathy?
Patient: Yes, I had bilateral retinopathy, planned for surgery next month.

Physician: So obviously you have poorly controlled, long lasting diabetes, with multiple micro vascular complications and you were offered Insulin before, but you didn't start it, can you give me a reason?
Patient: I hate needles, it's difficult for me to read and adjust the doses and I have no one to give me the injection.

The physician started to examine Mr. Ali.

On Examination:

Vital Signs are Normal
BMI=30
Local: No swelling or redness, +ve thickened waxy skin of both hands
Fixed flexion Deformity of Metacarpophalangeal and Proximal interphalangeal Joints bilateral.
Prayer Hand Sign +ve

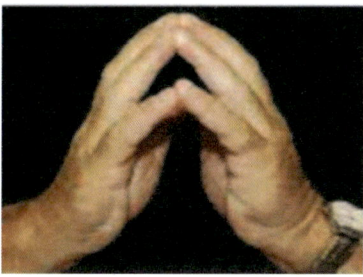

Figure 13: Prayer Hand Sign

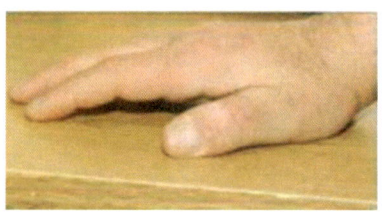

Figure 14: +ve Table Top Sign

Range of Motion: limitation in extension of proximal interphalangeal and metacarpophalangeal joints of both hands.

Tests for carpal tunnel syndrome; Tinel test -ve, Phalen test -ve, Carpal compression test -ve.

The physician ordered labs including Complete Blood Count, ESR, CRP, RF, Vitamin B12, HbA1C, and Urine Albumin/Creatinine Ratio.

Laboratory Exam:

Hb=12.5
CBC=N
ESR=n
CRP=n
VitD3=60
Vit B12=n
HbA1C=10 poorly controlled
UAC=8 elevated (micro albuminuria)
X-ray hands showed no skeletal deformity.

EMG nerve Conduction Study to rule out Carpal Tunnel Syndrome was -ve.

The Physician had a provisional diagnosis; Diabetic Stiff Hand Syndrome (Diabetic Cheiroarthropathy) plus worsening peripheral neuropathy related to poorly controlled Diabetes associated with microangiopathy (Peripheral neuropathy, Retinopathy, and Microalbuminuria)

The physician explained the condition to the patient and advised the patient to control his blood sugar in order to find improvement. He doubled the dose of gabapentin to target neuropathy. He referred the patient to Orthopedic Services for opinion and further management.

*Abbreviation Elaboration

* EMG: Electromyogram

References

1. Kim, H., Bialonczyk, D. and Goldman, J. (2016). Pointing Out the Facts: Diabetes Stiff Hand Syndrome (DSHS) | Well Life Medical. [online] https://www.welllifemedical.org/pointing-out-the-facts-diabetes-stiff-hand-syndrome-dshs/. Available at: https://www.welllifemedical.org/pointing-out-the-facts-diabetes-stiff-hand-syndrome-dshs/#:~:text=Diabetic%20stiff%20hand%20syndrome%20 (DSHS.
2. Goyal, A., Tiwari, V. and Gupta, Y. (2018). Diabetic Hand: A Neglected Complication of Diabetes Mellitus. Cureus, https://www.ncbi.nlm.nih.gov/pmc/issues/315353/(PMC6084697).
3. Limited Joint Mobility in Diabetes Mellitus: The Clinical Implications. (2011). www.rheumatologynetwork.com, [online] 28(4). Available at: https://www.rheumatologynetwork.com/view/limited-joint-mobility-diabetes-mellitus-clinical-implications [Accessed 14 Jan. 2022].

Dementia Chapter

Adil H. Alharthi, MD
Khalid A. Almutairi, MD

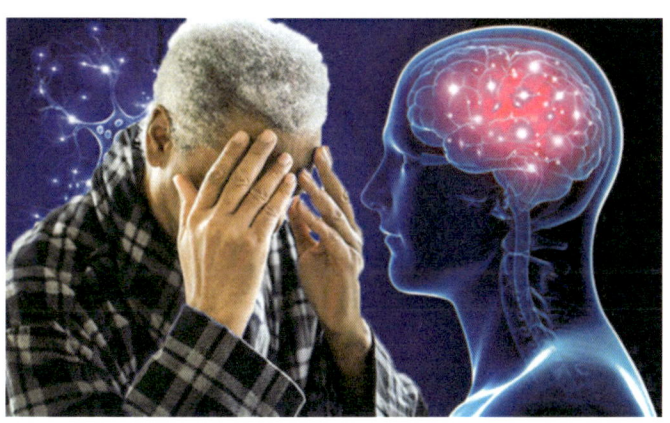

Case Study 1

An 80-year-old gentleman was brought after his family noticed him being forgetful.

Physician: Since when did you notice the forgetfulness?
The son: For the last month. Now, Dad doesn't remember anything we ask him about.

Physician: Who lives with Dad?
Son: He is living alone, but we visit him frequently.

Physician: Did you notice any fever, vomiting or diarrhea?
The son: No.

Physician: Did you notice any odd behavior in him lately?
The son: No.

Physician: What medications is he taking currently?
The son: I brought you his two medications for diabetes, and one medication for hypertension.

Physician notices Gliclazide, Glucophage and Co-Diovan
Physician: Dad needs to be seen by the neurologist.

Case Study 1 Ideal Scenario
Continued:

Physician: Since when was Dad living alone?
The son: About a month.

Physician: Is Dad still praying every day?
The son: Yes.

Physician: Did you see him praying yourself?
The son: Yes…

Physician: Do you need to remind him the Maghreb prayer is three rakaa and Ishaa prayer is four rakaa?
The son: No.

Physician: Next time please bring Dad so I can examine him. I think he may be having depression.

Junior Physician Mistakes:

- Impressions made exclusively according to the son's side of the story in spite of the son not living with the patient.
- Physician failed to notice that the onset of symptoms started at the same time of living alone.
- Physician needs to examine patients' memories of their strong beliefs like worshiping and prayer time.
- Physician needs to examine the patient for symptoms and signs of pseudodementia.

Clinical Pearls and Take-Home Messages

Pseudodementia, also known as depression-related cognitive dysfunction, is characterized by temporary declines in mental cognition. This term is applied to functional psychiatric conditions, such as depression and schizophrenia, which can mimic organic dementia but are essentially reversible with appropriate treatment.

Unlike dementia, which often develops gradually, pseudodementia typically manifests with a sudden and brief onset of disturbance. In clinical assessments, individuals with pseudodementia can be distinguished from those with true dementia when their memory is tested. Those with pseudodementia may respond by stating they are unsure of the answer, while still maintaining intact attention and concentration. Additionally, they may exhibit signs of distress. In contrast, individuals with true dementia may provide incorrect answers, display poor attention and concentration, and appear indifferent or unconcerned.

DEMENTIA	DEPRESSIVE PSEUDODEMENTIA
Progressive onset	Rapid onset
Long term symptomatology	Short term symptomatology
Mood variations	Consistently depressed mood
The patient tries to answer to the questions	Short answers like "I don't know", negativism
Patient is concealing amnesia	Highlighting amnesia
Constant cognitive decline	Fluctuating cognitive impairment

Table 8: Differential diagnosis between dementia and pseudodementia

References

1. Wikipedia. (2021). Pseudodementia. [online] Available at: https://en.wikipedia.org/wiki/Pseudodementia [Accessed 13 Jan. 2022].
2. www.encephalos.gr. (n.d.). Encephalos Journal. [online] Available at: http://www.encephalos.gr/48-3-07e.htm [Accessed 13 Jan. 2022].
3. Anon, (n.d.). Reversible Cognitive Disorder – Pseudodementia. [online] Available at: https://www.mentalhelp.net/cognitive-disorders/pseudodementia/ [Accessed 13 Jan. 2022].

Case Study 2

An 80-year-old lady came to the clinic after she started to wet her bed at night.

Physician: Since when did that start?
Patient: I think I first noticed it three days ago.

Physician: Do you have painful urination?
Patient: I think not.

Physician: Is your memory okay?
Patient's daughter: She started on a skin patch after the neurologist said she has dementia.

Physician: Can you tell me more about that please?
Patient's daughter: She was forgetting things. It is difficult for her to make decisions, and once she was walking and forgot where she was going.

Physician: I will make neurology and urology clinic appointments.

Case Study 2 Ideal Scenario

An 80-year-old lady came to the clinic after she started to wet her bed at night.

Physician: Since when did that start?
Patient: I think I first noticed it three days ago.

Physician: Do you have painful urination?
Patient: I think not.

Physician: Is your memory okay?

Patient's daughter: She was started on a skin patch after the neurologist said she has dementia.

Physician: Can you tell me more about that please?

Patient's daughter: She was forgetting things; it was difficult for her to make decisions and once she was walking and forgot where she was going.

Physician: Does Mom have other medications?

Patient's daughter: Yes, her diabetes and hypertensive pills. I brought them.

Physician: Who helps Mom with her meds.

Patient's daughter: She has always been taking care of her medications by herself.

Physician: Mom, can you show me how you take your medication?

Physician noticed the patient was struggling to read which medication she was holding and struggling to maintain a handgrip around it as well.

Patient's random blood sugar was found to be 20 mmol/L (high).

Junior Physician Mistakes:

- Physician wanted a fast fixed referral plan.
- Physician accepted the daughter's explanation despite she was not living with mom.
- Physician did not review the medications?
- Physician failed to put the patient's skills in handling the medication to the test.
- Physician considered three days as an acceptable duration of a new dementia related symptom.
- Failure to diagnose uncontrolled diabetes which is a potentially treatable condition.

Conclusion

Urinary incontinence secondary to uncontrolled diabetes due to poor vision (cannot read the medication label), frailty (cannot maintain a good hand grip) in a patient with underlying dementia.

Pearls and Take-Home Messages

Diabetes is predominantly a condition that individuals manage on their own, and leading up to a dementia diagnosis, most patients likely handle their blood sugar levels independently. Deteriorating glycemic control, missed appointments, or unexpected hypoglycemic incidents should alert healthcare providers to potential cognitive decline in these patients. Those with cognitive dysfunction may struggle to remember medication schedules, recognize hypo and hyperglycemia, and take corrective actions, deviating from the typical behavior expected of a diabetic patient without cognitive impairment. It is crucial for healthcare professionals to actively address the diagnosis of dementia and take a proactive approach to monitor these patients to ensure their well-being.

Another concern is the variability in nutritional intake and weight loss. As cognition declines and dementia advances, patients often experience a decrease in appetite and nutritional intake. This not only impacts choices and dosages of medications, particularly insulin, but also heightens the risk of hypoglycemic episodes. A recent study revealed a heightened risk of hypoglycemic incidents in dementia patients undergoing intensive management. Prolonged nutritional deficits leading to diminished glycogen stores in the liver further complicate the management of hypoglycemia, potentially predisposing individuals to severe episodes that require external assistance for recovery. This complication poses challenges in acute settings where intramuscular glucagon may not yield the desired effect.

The management of individuals with both diabetes and dementia demands careful consideration and continuous evaluation. Regular assessment should extend beyond just monitoring food intake to include the individual's capacity to administer medication appropriately. Additionally, this evaluation should encompass the needs and capabilities of the patient's caregivers.

References

1. Puttanna, A. and Padinjakara, N.K. (2017). Management of diabetes and dementia. British Journal of Diabetes, 17(3), p.93.
2. Bunn, F., Goodman, C., Malone, J.R., Jones, P.R., Burton, C., Rait, G., Trivedi, D., Bayer, A. and Sinclair, A. (2016). Managing diabetes in people with dementia: protocol for a realist review. Systematic Reviews, [online] 5(1). Available at: https://www.ncbi.nlm.nih.gov/pmc/articles/PMC4705581/.

Case Study 3

A Family Medicine Physician went with the Home Healthcare to the home of an 80-year-old gentleman who's known to have multi-comorbidities advanced dementia bedridden and totally dependent on his family for his activities of daily living.

The patient's son: Dad is different than he was in the last week.
Physician: What did you notice?

The patient's son: He's hitting his private nurse, spitting on her and cursing her every time she wants to help him. I brought another nurse but he treated her the same way.
Physician: Does Dad have a fever?
The patient's son: No

Physician: Any head trauma?
The patient's son: No.

Physician: Dad needs to be reviewed by the Psychiatrist.

Case Study 3 Ideal Scenario
A Family Medicine Physician went with the Home Healthcare to the home of an 80-year-old gentleman who's known to have multi-comorbidities, advanced dementia, bedridden and totally dependent on his family for his activities of daily living.

The patient's son: Dad is different than he was the last week.
Physician: What did you notice?

The patient's son: He's hitting his private nurse, spitting on her and cursing her every time she wants to help him. I brought another nurse but he treated her the same way.

Physician: Does Dad attack you when you try to help him?
The patient's son: No.

Physician: So, what does the nurse do that you don't?
The patient's son: She feeds him by his naso-gastric tube, she changes his diapers and she bathes him.

Physician and his nurse started feeding him by his NG tube. He started becoming aggressive to both of them then they attempted to change his diaper and found that he has fiery red rash around his inguinal folds that is very tender and made the patient more aggressive to them.

Physician: Dad has a diaper rash that becomes tender every time his diapers are changed; he needs ointments for that.

One month after the diaper rash improved the patient's aggressiveness improved as well.

Junior Physician Mistakes:

- He didn't examine the patient.
- Any new onset symptom needs proper investigation for causes.
- He didn't try to find out if the aggressiveness is directed against one person or one place to discover the appropriate precipitating factors.

Conclusion

Behavioral and Psychological Symptoms of Dementia (BPSD) manifested as aggression.

Clinical Pearls and Take-Home Messages

- The phrase "Behavioral and Psychological Symptoms of Dementia (BPSD)" encompasses a range of non-cognitive and non-neurological symptoms associated with dementia, including agitation, aggression, psychosis, depression, and apathy. BPSD is encountered in at least 80% of individuals with dementia.
- It is crucial to gather a comprehensive history and conduct a thorough clinical examination involving both the patient and their family or care team. To formulate a personalized treatment plan, it is advisable to create a therapeutic decision tree that considers the individual's unique characteristics and their environmental risk profile.

References

1. bpac.org.nz. (n.d.). Managing the Behavioural and Psychological Symptoms of Dementia – bpacnz. [online] Available at: https://bpac.org.nz/2020/bpsd.aspx.
2. Tible, O.P., Riese, F., Savaskan, E. and von Gunten, A. (2017). Best practice in the management of behavioural and psychological symptoms of dementia. Therapeutic Advances in Neurological Disorders, [online] 10(8), pp.297–309. Available at: https://www.ncbi.nlm.nih.gov/pmc/articles/PMC5518961/

Case Study 4

A Family Medicine Physician went with the Home Healthcare to the home of an 80-year-old gentleman who's known to have multi-comorbidities, advanced dementia, bedridden and totally dependent on his family for his activities of daily living.

The patient's son: Dad has been ill since I passed by the last 3 days.
Physician: What did you notice?

The patient's son: He's very hot, vomiting and not as responding as his usual.

The physician examines the patient with his nurse. The patient is lying flat. He is awake and attentive but not responding. He looks ill, sweaty, he is breathing comfortably but with fever, his arms and legs are stiff with hypertonia all over.

Physician: Dad needs to be shifted to hospital urgently.

In ER Medications reviewed and the patient is found to be on antipsychotics for a week for aggressiveness and insomnia related to his BPSD.
Patient is suspected of having Neuroleptic Malignant Syndrome.
Admitted under Medicine and seen by Psychiatry.

Junior Physician Mistakes:
· Physician noticed that it was an emergency and acted accordingly but failed to review the medications and the medication history.
· Comorbid patients need detailed assessment that includes drug to drug and drug to disease interactions and overdose complications as well.

Clinical Pearls and Take-Home Messages

Neuroleptic malignant syndrome (NMS) is an infrequent yet potentially life-threatening abnormal reaction to neuroleptic medications. It manifests with symptoms such as fever, muscle stiffness, altered mental status, and dysfunction of the autonomic nervous system. NMS typically emerges shortly after starting neuroleptic treatment or following a dosage increase.

Diagnosing NMS involves confirming recent use of neuroleptic drugs (within the last 1-4 weeks), observing hyperthermia (body temperature exceeding 38°C), and identifying muscular rigidity, accompanied by at least five of the following: changes in mental status, rapid heart rate, and either high or low blood pressure.

Complications associated with neuroleptic malignant syndrome encompass issues like dehydration due to reduced oral intake, acute kidney failure resulting from muscle breakdown (rhabdomyolysis), and the development of deep vein thrombosis and pulmonary embolism due to muscle rigidity and immobility. It's important to note that refraining from antipsychotic use can lead to complications stemming from unmanaged psychosis.

References

1. Neuroleptic Malignant Syndrome: Practice Essentials, Background, Pathophysiology. (2021). eMedicine. [online] Available at: https://emedicine.medscape.com/article/816018-overview.
2. www.medscape.com. (n.d.). How is neuroleptic malignant syndrome (NMS) diagnosed? [online] Available at: https://www.medscape.com/answers/816018-101130/how-is-neuroleptic-malignant-syndrome-nms-diagnosed [Accessed 13 Jan. 2022].
3. www.medscape.com. (n.d.). What are the complications of neuroleptic malignant syndrome (NMS)? [online] Available at: https://www.medscape.com/answers/816018-101119/what-are-the-complications-of-neuroleptic-malignant-syndrome-nms [Accessed 13 Jan. 2022].

Case Study 5

Ali is an 85-year-old male, known case of dementia, presented to Family Medicine with his son and brother. They noticed that he is disoriented, cannot remember things and agitated.

Physician: For how long has your father been like that?
The son: For many years but it increased recently.

Physician: Is there any other complaint?
The son: My father is not paying attention to us when we talk to him in the last three days.

Physician: You know these changes can happen with old age; your father needs to be referred to neurology.

What went wrong in this scenario?
Physician assumed that the patient's condition deteriorated due to the natural history of dementia.
Physician missed that this is a case of delirium on top of dementia.
Physician mismanaged the case endangering patient life.

Ideal Scenario

Ali is an 85-year-old male, presented to Family Medicine with his son and brother. They noticed that he is disoriented, cannot remember things and agitated.

Physician: For how long has your father been like that?

The son: For many years, but it increased recently.

Physician: Does your father have feeding difficulties, diarrhea, vomiting, Trauma, dysuria or fever?

The son: I have noticed that he is screaming and pointing to his urethra upon urination?

Physician: What medication is he on?
The son: Some tablets for diabetes and dementia.

Physician: We will do urinalysis and culture.

Physician: Urine dipstick is positive for leukocyte and nitrite, I think your father is having a urinary tract infection, I will prescribe him the proper treatment, and he will be okay to revisit me within three days.

DSM-5 Diagnostic Criteria for Delirium

A. A disturbance in attention (i.e., reduced ability to direct, focus, sustain, and shift attention) and awareness (reduced orientation to the environment).
B. The disturbance develops over a short period of time (usually hours to a few days), represents a change from baseline attention and awareness, and tends to fluctuate in severity during the course of a day.
C. An additional disturbance in cognition (e.g., memory deficit, disorientation, language, visuo-spatial ability, or perception).
D. The disturbances in Criteria A and C are not explained by another preexisting, established, or evolving neurocognitive disorder and do not occur in the context of a severely reduced level of arousal, such as commas.
E. There is no evidence from the history, physical examination, or laboratory findings that the disturbance is a direct physiological consequence of another medical condition, substance intoxication or withdrawal (i.e., due to a drug of abuse or to a medication), or exposure to a toxin, or is due to multiple etiologies.

Clinical Evaluation

Evaluation should be individualized based on the patient's chief concern, medical history, current illness, and physical examination findings. Although imaging is not generally indicated, computed tomography of the head is recommended for patients presenting with new focal neurologic deficits, history of head trauma, or fever associated with encephalopathy. If seizures are suspected, or if the cause of delirium is unclear, electroencephalography should be considered.

Basic Workup for Delirium

All older persons presenting with delirium require a basic workup including a complete blood count, measurement of electrolyte levels, renal and liver panel, urinalysis, and electrocardiography.

Medical and Psychiatric Events Requiring Urgent Evaluation.

Medical Issues:

Dramatic change in vital signs with associated signs and symptoms:

- systolic blood pressure less than 90 mm Hg;
- heart-rate less than 50 beats per minute or greater than 120 beats per minute.
- respirations greater than 30 breaths per minute;
- temperature less than 96°F (36°C) or greater than 101°F (38°C)
- New-onset focal deficits.
- New-onset respiratory distress, with increasing hypoxia and dyspnea.
- Signs of a serious underlying condition causing delirium (e.g., stroke, chest pain, hematuria).

Psychiatric or Behavioral Issues:

Escalating physically aggressive behavior or threats of violence persistent danger to self or others.

References

1. Kalish VB, Gillham JE, Unwin BK. Delirium in older persons: evaluation and management. Am Fam Physician. 2014; 90(3):150-8.
2. American Psychiatric Association. Diagnostic and Statistical Manual of Mental Disorders. 5th ed. Washington, DC: American Psychiatric Association; 2013.

Blue Mood Chapter

Adnan A. Mufti, MD
Nayef A. Aljohani, MD

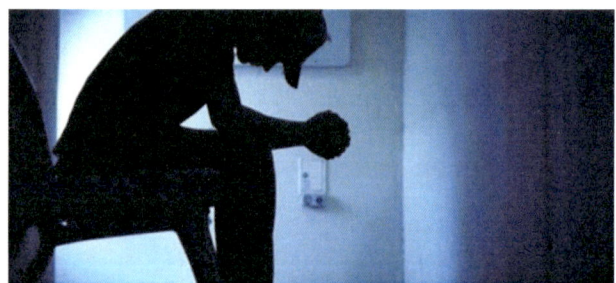

Case Study 1

Missing asking for manic/hypomanic symptoms
Missing asking for past psychiatric Hx

Sara is a 25-year-old single lady who was brought by her mother to the clinic.

She is a university student studying English language. She is the eldest between her two sisters. Her mother noticed she is eating very little over the past months & her clothes seems loose on her lately. She stays most of the times in her room and crying. She even missed attending few lectures & does not seem to be concerned about it. During the interview Sarah seemed uninterested & hardly talking.

Physician: Do you have any stomach problem?
Patient: No.

Physician: Do you have any psychological problem?
Patient: No answer.

Physician: Tell me what seems to be the problem?
Patient: No answer.

Physician: Proceeds to physical examination and finds nothing significant other than looking tired.

Ideal Scenario

Sara is a 25-year-old single lady who was brought by her mother to the clinic.

She is a university student studying English language. She is the eldest between her two sisters. Her mother noticed she is eating very little over the past months and her clothes seems loose on her lately. She stays most of the times in her room crying. She even missed attending few lectures and does not seem to be concerned about it. During the interview Sarah seemed uninterested and hardly talking.

Physician: Hello Sarah, your mother sound very concerned about you and I'm going to do my best to help you. Can you tell me what happened over the past month changed you?

Patient: Hesitant at the start but answered, "I don't enjoy being with people as before and feeling down most of the time."

Physician: You look tired. How is your sleep?
Patient: I have difficulty sleeping.

Physician: Your mother noticed you eat very little and possibly lost some weight. Tell me about that.
Patient: I lost my appetite.

Physician: And you missed a few of your lectures, how did that happen?
Patient: I just don't care about it anymore. I didn't feel like going.

Junior Physician Mistakes:

- Physician did not approach the patient in an empathic way.
- Failed to establish good rapport with the patient.
- Using open ended questions to get more details.

Case 1 Continued:

Physician: Did you have any death wishes or suicidal thoughts?
Patient: Sometimes I wished I was dead.

Physician: Have you experienced any hallucinations or abnormal experience over the past month?
Patient: No.

Physician: Have you ever had such symptoms before?

Patient: No.

What is the proper diagnosis?
A. Adjustment disorder
B. Major depressive disorder
C. Bipolar disorder
D. Schizophrenia

Mother reported Sarah did not have similar symptoms before, but recalls a year ago she noticed a period of about a week when she was more energetic & active, increased talk and an exaggerated sense of humor which annoyed her professor at the university, they did not think it was something significant as it disappeared afterwards.

Junior Physician Mistakes of the Previous Section:
Always ask about manic/hypomanic symptoms when assessing depressive symptoms as part of the present illness or past psychiatric history.
Physician failed to pick up bipolar disorder.

Case 1 Continued:
Physician: Sarah, you suffer from a psychiatric illness called (bipolar disorder) and currently you have a depressive episode, we need to start treatment so you can improve and enjoy your life again.

Patient: Is it possible that I may get well?
Physician: Yes, bipolar disorder is a treatable condition. I will prescribe an anti-depressant medication and give you a follow up appointment after two weeks.

Sarah comes in after 2 weeks with her mother, she is irritable, argumentative and feeling energetic although sleeping only 2-3 hours for the past week.

Junior Physician Mistakes of the Previous Section:
- In bipolar depression prescribing anti-depressant medication alone will cause the patient to developed manic/hypomanic symptoms.
- Adding a mood stabilizer or antipsychotic medication to the antidepressant medication is advisable.

Case Study 2

Missing substance use

Mr. Saeed is a 46-year-old married gentleman, who came to the clinic by himself complaining of difficulty to sleep and poor concentration, he reported recently having warnings from work for being late and multiple conflicts with colleagues. He is hypertensive and stable on his medications.

Physician: For how long have you had these complaints?
Mr. Saeed: Recently over the past two weeks, but I had them on & off for many years, I noticed it being worse the past year.

Physician: Do you have any other complaints?
Mr. Saeed: Yes, I feel tired and don't want to do anything. My wife complains that I'm neglecting my house responsibilities.

Physician: Tell me, Mr. Saeed, how is your mood? Do you enjoy company of your family & friends?
Mr. Saeed: Honestly speaking, I feel down and started to avoid them. I want to stay alone all the time.
Physician: I believe that you suffer from a depressive disorder. Mr. Saeed, I will prescribe an anti-depressant for you. You will be fine over few weeks.
Mr. Saeed follows up after two months with no much improvement in his symptoms even on reaching the maximum dose of antidepressant medications, in fact his sleep became worse and his blood pressure is on the higher side.

Physician: It seems the antidepressant I prescribed did not help you, we have to change to another type of antidepressant medication.

Ideal Case 2 Scenario

Mr. Saeed is a 46-year-old married gentleman, who came to the clinic by himself complaining of difficulty to sleep and poor concentration. He reported recently having warnings from work for being late and multiple conflicts with colleagues. He is hypertensive and stable on his medications. The physician confirmed symptoms of a depressive disorder.

Physician: Mr. Saeed, do you have another medical illness other than hypertension?
Mr. Saeed: None.

Physician: Do you take any medication other than the anti-hypertensive treatment, or use any recreational drug?
Mr. Saeed: Well doctor, because of the work load I use sometimes things like (Adderall/Ritalin) to keep my energy up, and it helps to have a better mood.
Physician: Mr. Saeed, these medications actually worsen your symptoms and probably the main cause of your complaints. It raises your blood pressure. I recommend you to stop taking them and I will prescribe you an antidepressant medication. I recommend that you see a psychiatrist as well for more professional advice.

Junior Physician Mistakes:

- Physician did not inquire about medical illnesses/illicit drugs and substances of abuse that may contribute to depression.
- Physician jumped to conclude that antidepressant was ineffective & prescribed another antidepressant medication before reviewing the diagnosis.
- Better to refer to a psychiatrist in complicated cases.

Case Study 3

Postpartum Depression, Missing Safety Assessment:

Mrs. Aljameel is a 28-year-old lady who delivered her first baby two weeks ago after a full term pregnancy by SVD. She was brought to the clinic accompanied by her husband as he noticed his wife crying, fearful & unable to sleep for the past 10 days. Lately she could hardly care for her new baby or herself.

Physician: How was the pregnancy period and delivery?
Husband: It went well and uneventful mostly, but during the last days of pregnancy I noticed her a bit nervous and preferred to sit alone.

Physician: Has any new events or stressors develop other than the delivery?
Husband: Nothing.

Physician: Mrs. Aljameel, is there something bothering you recently although I expected you to be happy that you are a new mom?
Mrs. Aljameel: I don't know doctor, I just feel down, I'm not enjoying my motherhood. I'm afraid I may not be a good mom. I keep thinking something bad may happen to the baby. This is a big burden that I can't handle.
Mrs. Aljameel became tearful and weepy.

Physician: But I'm sure your husband and all the family will be glad to help you and support you in this.
Husband: Yes, the whole family is happy with the baby and willing to lend a hand.
Mrs. Aljameel: No, it's useless. I can't burden them with all this. Everybody has their own life.
Physician: Did you ever experience any unusual voices you heard or images you saw over the past weeks (auditory/visual hallucinations)?

Mrs. Aljameel: No, Doctor.

Physician: Okay, Mrs. Aljameel. I believe you are suffering from a major depression with postpartum onset (postpartum depression). I will prescribe an antidepressant medication, and I expect you to start to improve over the coming few weeks.

Physician: The medication is excreted in the breast milk in very minimal amounts which will not harm the baby, especially if the mother pumps out the breast milk before the medication dose then she can feed it to the baby later on when he is hungry, or if you are worried she can start bottle feeds as it's very important to take the medication.

What is the most proper management?
A. Start an antidepressant treatment.
B. Start an anxiolytic treatment.
C. Start an antidepressant treatment with a small dose of an antipsychotic.
D. Take more details of psychotic symptoms and safety assessment.

After few days the baby is rushed to the hospital emergency room as the husband came from work and saw his wife attempting to strangulate the baby with the pillow.

Ideal Case 3 Scenario

Mrs. Aljameel is a 28-year-old lady who delivered her first baby two weeks ago after a full term pregnancy by SVD. She was brought to the clinic accompanied by her husband as he noticed his wife crying, fearful, and unable to sleep for the past 10 days. Lately, she could hardly care for her new baby or herself.

Physician: Asking all the detailed questions about depressive symptoms. (As mentioned above).

Physician: Did you ever experience any unusual voices you heard or images you saw over the past weeks? (Auditory/visual hallucinations)
Mrs. Aljameel: No doctor.

Physician: Mrs. Aljameel, how do you feel toward your baby?

Mrs. Aljameel: I have no much emotions toward him as I expected, for this I'm more guilty.

Physician: Do you ever have any thoughts to harm yourself, Mrs. Aljameel?

Mrs. Aljameel: No answer.

Physician: Do you ever think you want to just get rid of the baby or may harm him?

Mrs. Aljameel Answering in tears: I do have such thoughts at times. I believe he will have a miserable life for which I want to spare him all the pain in life.

Physician: Empathically talks to the husband and wife. Okay, I believe Mrs. Aljameel is suffering from a major depression with psychotic features with postpartum onset and under these symptoms there is a risk to the baby's safety, I will refer her to the psychiatric service urgently for a specialist opinion and I'm confident they will provide the best management.

Junior Physician Mistakes:

During assessment for mood disorders always inquire about psychotic symptoms.

Psychotic symptoms are not only different types of hallucinations, it includes delusional thoughts as well.

Never miss safety assessment (risk of harm to self or others) and refer urgently to the specialized psychiatric service if present.

Case Study 4

Missing Asking About the Stressors and The Duration of Symptoms:

Nada is 20-year-old female, she is married, lives with her husband, has a two-year-old boy. She is a university student, she is complaining of anxiety and is worrying of the future, she is worried about her performance in the university and also worried about her family, she had difficulty paying attention in class and finishing her assignment. she often feels restless, is spending long periods of time alone in her room crying and feeling overwhelmed, she reported she had trouble falling asleep at night, there was no family history of mental or physical illnesses.

Physician: Hello Nada, I'm going to help you, can you tell me about your anxiety and worries?

Patient: I am worrying about my health, my family's health and my performance in the university, I feel I am overwhelmed of thinking.

Physician: Do you feel you can't stop worrying?

Patient: Yes.

Physician: What about your sleep tell me more?

Patient: I have difficulty falling asleep.

Physician: You told me that you are crying most of the time, tell me more.

Patient: Yes, I feel sad and I want to cry.

Physician: Did you have any death wishes or suicidal thoughts?

Patient: No, I didn't.

Physician: Have you ever had such symptoms before?
Patient: No.

What is the proper diagnosis?
A. Major depressive disorder
B. Generalized anxiety disorder.
C. Adjustment disorder.
D. Bipolar disorder.

Case 4 Continued:

Physician: Nada, you suffer from a psychiatric illness called Generalized Anxiety Disorder, we need to start treatment so you can improve & enjoy your life again.

Patient: Okay.
Physician: I will prescribe an anti-depressant medication which treats anxiety as well and psychotherapy and give you a follow up appointment after three weeks.

Patient went to another senior physician for second opinion.

The senior physician asked her about the cause of her worries and she said she moved to a new city five months ago with her husband and son, and this city is far from her parents and she entered a new university there.

The senior physician advised her with psychotherapy sessions which provide emotional support and help her to get back to her normal routine and teach her coping skills to deal with stressful events.

Patient improved with psychotherapy sessions.

Junior Physician Mistakes:
- Physician failed to pick up the diagnosis (adjustment disorder).

Always ask about the stressors and duration of symptoms when assessing adjustment disorder.

Clinical Pearls and Take-Home messages

- Adjustment disorder always triggered by traumatic events such as the death of loved one or loss of job or moving away from home (moved to other city).
- People with GAD suffering from long and consistent history of having anxiety, people with adjustment disorder only experience the symptoms in times of stress or change and there is a significant improvement in their anxiety once they adapt to a life change.

References

1. Sadock, B. J, Virginia Alcott Sadock, Pedro Ruiz (2015) Kaplan and Sadock's Synopsis of psychiatry: Behavioral sciences/clinical psychiatry. 11th edn. Philadelphia: Lippincott Williams & Wilkins.
2. American Psychiatric Association (2014). DSM-5 TM guidebook the essential companion to the Diagnostic and statistical manual of mental disorders, fifth edition. Washington, Dc American Psychiatric Publishing.
3. National Institute for Health and Clinical Excellence, 2012. Clinical case scenarios: Common mental health disorders in primary care. NHS, Manchester.

Lower Limb Edema Chapter

Adil H. Alharthi, MD
Khalid A. Almutairi, MD

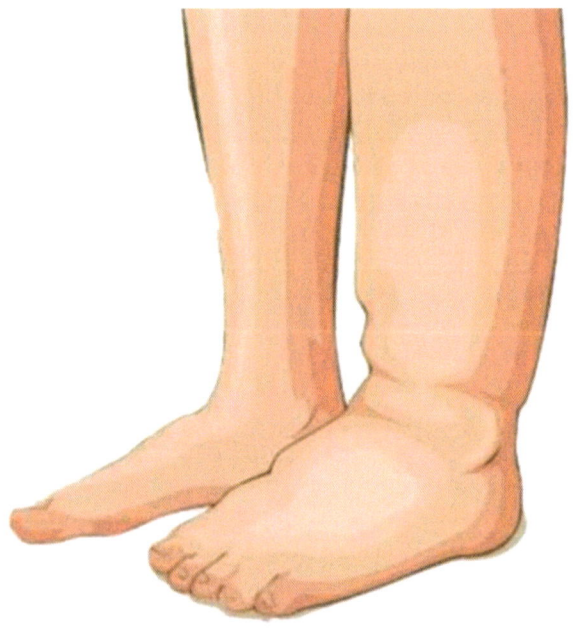

Case Study 1

A 70-year-old man presented with lower limb swelling and an abdominal ultra sound showing fatty liver.

Physician: Since when the lower limb started swelling?
Patient: A couple of weeks.

Physician: Do you drink alcohol?
Patient: Occasionally.

Physician: Did you receive blood transfusion in the past?
Patient: No.

Physician: Do you inject recreational drugs?
Patient: No.

Physician: You noticed fatigability and tiredness as well?
Patient: Yes.

Physician: You noticed reduced appetite as well?
Patient: Yes.

What is the proper diagnosis?
A. Liver cirrhosis
B. Congestive heart failure
C. Plural effusion for investigation
D. All of the above

Case Study 1 Ideal Scenario

A 70-year-old man presented with lower limb swelling and a liver ultra sound showed fatty liver.

Physician: Since when is the lower limb swelling?
Patient: A couple of weeks.

Physician: Can you elaborate more about that?
Patient: Now even taking two tabs of diuretics twice daily does not help with the leg swelling.

Physician: Can I ask who advised you to take the diuretic two tabs twice daily.
Patient: My cardiologist I missed follow up with him since the Covid pandemic.

Physician: Can you tell me more about your heart issues?
Patient: I underwent a Coronary Artery Bypass Grafting CABG ten years ago. Symptoms improved at first, but deteriorated later a year ago, so they did a Coronary angioplasty and left a stent in my artery. Things got better, but it started worsening in the last weeks.

Physician: Can you elaborate on the symptoms, which started worsening?
Patient: I still lose my breath when I walk, but lately I started to lose my breath even when I am lying down.

What was the mistakes in the first scenario?

A. Physician used leading questions* in the beginning of the history.
B. Physician didn't give appropriate time to patient to elaborate his concerns.
C. Physician was biased by the liver ultra sound result.
D. All of the Above

Clinical Pearls and Take-Home Messages

1. Diagnosis shouldn't be formulated before proper history and examination.
2. In the case of a common presenting symptom (e.g., shortness of breath, palpitation or abdominal pain) diagnosis should be accepted only after ruling out the differential diagnosis.
3. Labs and radiological investigations are subjected to be false positive or false negative so its significance should be determined in the context of the history and physical examination.

Case Study 2

A 70-year-old woman presenting with leg swelling on examination. There is redness and swelling. Echo done two months ago shows an EF of 70% no wall motion abnormalities and normal valve function. Patient referred immediately to ER. (Figure 1-1)

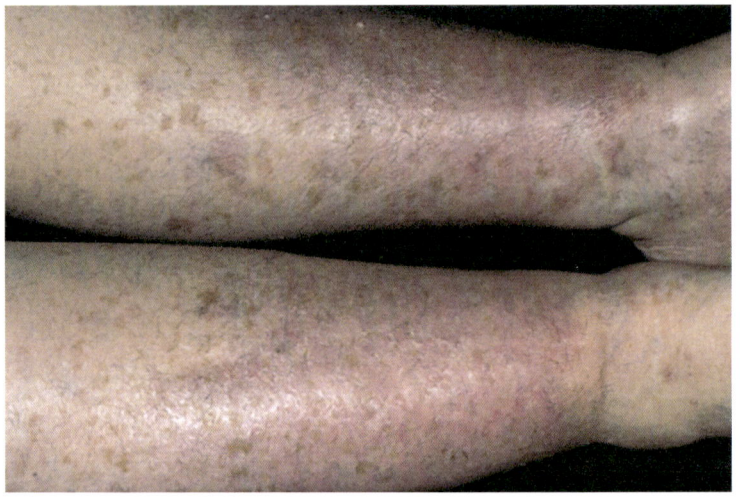

Figure 15: showing Lower Limbs rash

What is the appropriate diagnosis?

A. Cellulitis
B. DVT
C. Lymphatic obstruction
D. Stasis dermatitis
E. Others

Case Study 2 Continued

A 70-year-old woman presented with leg swelling on examination there is redness and swelling.

Physician: Since when is the redness?
Patient: Noticed a couple of weeks ago.

Physician: Is it unilateral or bilateral?
Patient: It is bilateral.

Physician: Is the redness fiery or dusky red?
Patient: Dusky red (in keeping with chronicity)

Physician: Is the redness tender or not?
Patient: No.

Physician: Are there other symptoms associated with LL Swelling?
Patient: I have exertional shortness of breath and fatigability.

The physician finds that her ECG shows failure of progression of R waves in chest leads with Q waves in inferior leads.

What was the potential mistakes in the first scenario?

- The normal ECHO biased the physician (Congestive Heart Failure is a clinical diagnosis and normal ECHO doesn't rule it out – Diastolic dysfunction)
- Physician was biased by redness (redness description and duration are in keeping with Status dermatitis which is common in Chronic Heart failure)
- Physician needed to rule out Cellulitis (redness being bilateral non-tender chronic and dusky red in color makes it unlikely to be Cellulitis – mostly Status dermatitis)

Pearls and Take-Home Massages:

Stasis dermatitis is a chronic condition characterized by inflammation, itching, and the development of ulcers on the lower legs. This condition commonly affects individuals with underlying issues that impact blood circulation in the legs, including chronic venous insufficiency, varicose veins, deep vein thrombosis (DVT), and congestive heart failure.

Heart failure with preserved ejection fraction (HFpEF) occurs when the left ventricle, the lower chamber of the heart, struggles to adequately fill with blood during the diastolic (filling) phase. This results in a reduced amount of blood being pumped out to the body, a condition also known as diastolic heart failure.

Case Study 3

An 80-year-old man known to have DM, HTN, GERD, IHD, Osteoporosis and Chronic Lymphocytic Leukemia presented with leg swelling.

Physician: Since when?
Patient: Noticed a couple of weeks ago.

Physician: When did you stop taking your medications?
Patient: I never stopped taking my medication.

Physician: Are you still compliant to dietary restriction?
Patient: Yes.

Physician: Are you still compliant to the daily exercise advice?
Patient: Yes.

Physician: What about dates? You are still eating that in the afternoon.
Patient: No.

What is the most likely cause of this patient leg swelling?

A. Nephrotic syndrome
B. Congestive Heart Failure (CHF)
C. Diabetic autonomic neuropathy
D. Malignancy
E. Drug induced
F. All of the Above

Case 3 Corrected

An 80-year-old man known to have DM, HTN, GERD, IHD, Osteoporosis and Chronic Lymphocytic Leukemia presented with Leg swelling.

Physician: Since when?
Patient: Noticed a couple of weeks ago.

Physician: Can you elaborate more on that please?
Patient: I think it started after I did not find my physician due to the Covid pandemic and another physician saw me and prescribed different medications.

Physician: You seem to be compliant to your medications.
Patient: I try as much as I can.

Physician: What did you notice about the new medications?
Patient: After he prescribed the new medications, I started noticing leg swelling.

Physician: That is an excellent notice from you. Can you show me which medications were changed please?
Patient: It is this insulin injection once daily, and this HTN medication once daily as well.
Physician sees long-acting insulin (Glargine) and anti HTN (Amlodipine).

What was the potential mistakes in the first scenario?
A. Physician was biased by many non-compliant patients seen before
B. Physician is trying to prove his point of noncompliance to the patient (Confrontation History)
C. Patient responding on what will stop the confrontation questions (Lack of trust)
D. Physician is not familiar on Clerking Elder Multi comorbidity patient (Multi comorbidity taboo*)

Clinical Pearls and Take-Home Messages

• "Comorbidity" refers to the simultaneous presence of two or more chronic conditions within an individual, and it has distinct implications for safety considerations in primary care.

• Ensuring the safety of patients across their healthcare interactions is influenced by various challenges that arise based on the stages of life or the comprehensive health needs from birth to end-of-life. Individuals dealing with multiple health conditions present a specific and ongoing challenge to patient safety throughout their entire life cycle.

Patients with Multi-Morbidity Are at Higher Risk of Safety Issues for Many Reasons, Including:

• Polypharmacy, potentially resulting in reduced medication adherence and the occurrence of adverse drug events.

• Complicated management routines contribute to more frequent and intricate engagements with healthcare services, increasing the vulnerability to breakdowns in care delivery and coordination.

• Clear communication and patient-centered care are essential due to the intricate requirements of patients with complex needs.

• The necessity for vigilant self-management routines and the presence of competing priorities.

Case Study 4

A 51-year-old male with a history of HTN, DM and chronic alcohol abuse presenting with lower extremity swelling. He noticed one month of progressive, bilateral lower extremity swelling. In the past two weeks, no pain neither redness. He denies fevers/chills, chest pain, or shortness of breath. He also denies orthopnea and paroxysmal nocturnal dyspnea, although he did notice frequent daytime sleepiness.

What is the most likely cause of this patient's leg swelling?

A. Liver cirrhosis
B. Congestive heart failure
C. Cellulitis
D. DVT
E. Others

Physical Exam showed BMI 36, normal vital signs, no jaundice, normal breathing and heart sounds, JVP is 4 cm above sternal angle; liver is palpable 1 cm below costal margin. His lower extremities swollen bilaterally extending from ankles to mid-shin. Mild tenderness to palpation.

What is the most likely cause of this patient's leg swelling?

A. Liver cirrhosis
B. Congestive heart failure
C. Cellulitis
D. DVT
E. Others

His labs showed normal WBC, Creatinine, Albumin and BNP. The venous lower extremity ultrasound proved no DVT but there is a pulsatile flow in bilateral EIV (external iliac veins) suggestive of elevated right heart pressure.

What investigation you will do to confirm the diagnosis?

A. Echocardiogram
B. Pelvic and abdominal CT
C. Polysomnography
D. Lower limb venogram
E. Lymphoscintigraphy
F. A and B
G. A and C

Answers

Given the evidence of obesity, frequent daytime sleepiness, and ultrasound findings of pulsatile flow in external iliac veins indicate raised Rt side heart pressure which highly raise the suspicion of pulmonary hypertension caused by Obstructive Sleep Apnea. Echocardiogram and Polysomnography needed to confirm the diagnosis

Chronic bilateral lower extremity edema likely secondary to RT sided Heart failure arising from the pulmonary hypertension. In this case, there is no stigmata of cirrhosis and normal albumin, normal creatinine. Also, no evidence of DVT on ultrasound. Bilateral cellulitis also unlikely as the patient is afebrile without leukocytosis.

Clinical Pearls and Take-Home Messages

- Avoid falling in Availability Heuristics (bias)
- Availability Heuristics (biases) are mental shortcuts that relies on immediate examples that come to a given person's mind when evaluating a specific topic, concept, method, or decision.
- It is a bias in which the sub conscious fills in the gaps of knowledge and experience.

- In the above case (1), the physician thought about a diagnosis that he knows and is comfortable investigating and managing, so most questions are guided to fulfill his diagnosis.

How to prevent falling in the Availability Heuristics pitfall?

A. Use open ended questions in the beginning of the history.
B. Encourage the patient to reveal his concerns.
C. Spend more time exploring the symptom rather than pinpointing the diagnosis.
D. Avoid directing questions in relation to a lab or image finding early in the History (Labs could be false positive so it must be explored after a bias free proper history).
E. Don't be biased by the ECHO or CT finding (Ventricular dysfunction patient can present with other diagnosis).
F. Try to follow up the patient's progress by asking your colleagues (to learn from your mistakes and prevent repeating them).
G. Make your primary concern to help the patient as much as you can (not to find the appropriate diagnosis or to challenge him on needs of labs or referrals).

Apply the recommendations for assessing multi co-morbidity patients which are:

A. Prioritize what you want to accomplish during this office visit.
B. Ask patients for their concerns, goals, values, and preferences for a plan of action.
C. Communicate in simple language, avoid jargon*, and elicit understanding.
D. Collaborate with the interdisciplinary care team.
E. Coordinate care with caregiver and/or family.
F. Gain patients trust by motivating them for their notes and achievements.
G. Employ an evidence-based approach in creating a management plan.
H. Understand their social and financial challenges.
I. Understand it is common for the Multi co-morbidity patients to have psychological findings esp. depression.

Clinical Pearls of Lower Extremity Edema

• When gathering a patient's history, it's essential to note the timing of edema, its responsiveness to changes in position, and whether it's unilateral or bilateral. Additionally, assess medication history and screen for systemic diseases.
• Edema often results from a combination of factors.
• Rapid identification of causes requiring urgent intervention, such as deep vein thrombosis and heart failure, is crucial in cases of leg edema.
• Bilateral or generalized swelling may indicate systemic issues like congestive heart failure (especially right-sided), pulmonary hypertension, chronic renal or hepatic conditions (leading to hypoalbuminemia), protein-losing enteropathies, or severe malnutrition.
• Acute limb swelling within 72 hours is more indicative of conditions like deep venous thrombosis (DVT), cellulitis, ruptured popliteal cyst, or acute compartment syndrome from trauma.
• Certain medications, including calcium channel blockers, prednisone, and anti-inflammatory drugs, can induce edema as an adverse effect.
• Effective skin care is vital for preventing skin breakdown and venous ulcers. The management of eczematous (stasis) dermatitis involves the use of emollients and topical steroid creams.
• During the physical examination, assess for systemic causes of edema such as heart failure (e.g., jugular venous distention, crackles), renal disease (e.g., proteinuria, oliguria), hepatic disease (e.g., jaundice, ascites, asterixis), or thyroid disease (e.g., exophthalmos, tremor, weight loss). Evaluate edema for characteristics like pitting, tenderness, and skin changes.
• In cases of bilateral leg edema without clinical indications of heart failure or venous stasis, consider the following recommended laboratory investigations:

1. Complete blood count with platelet count.
2. Urinary protein and plasma creatinine.
3. Plasma potassium and sodium.
4. ALT (as liver disease is common in alcoholics).
5. TSH, especially if edema is present in areas other than the legs and does not exhibit pitting.
6. Fasting blood glucose.
7. Serum albumin (levels below 20 g/l often contribute to edema).

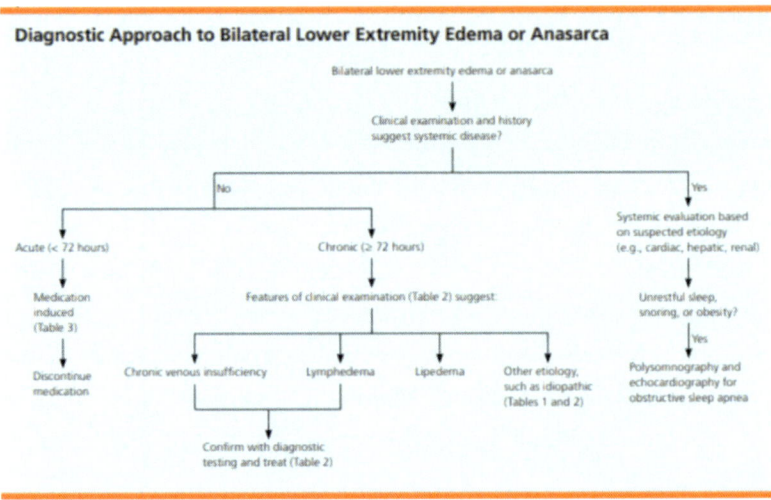

Figure 16: Algorithm for the Diagnosis of Bilateral Lower Extremity Edema

Definitions:

* Leading questions: Questions that prompts or encourages the answers wanted.
* Multi comorbidity taboo: Healthcare providers reluctant to assess or manage multi-comorbidity patient due to the multiple potential challenges they represent.
* Jargon: Special words or expressions used by a profession or group that are difficult for others to understand.

References

1. Trayes, K. and Studdiford, J. (2013). Edema: Diagnosis and Management. [online] 88(2). Available at: https://www.aafp.org/afp/2013/0715/afp20130715p102.pdf.
2. Editor (2014). Differential Diagnosis of Lower Extremity Edema. [online] Differential Diagnosis of. Available at: https://ddxof.com/lower-extremity-edema/ [Accessed 14 Jan. 2022].
3. Editors (n.d.). Leg oedema. [online] EBM Guidelines. Available at: https://www.ebm-guidelines.com/ebmg/ltk.free?p_artikkeli=ebm00099.

4. Multimorbidity Technical Series on Safer Primary Care. (n.d.). [online] Available at: https://apps.who.int/iris/bitstream/handle/10665/252275/9789241511650-eng.pdf?sequence=1.

Palpitation Chapter

Abdulrahim M. Basendwah, MD
Salem A. Assiri, MD
Suhair A. Al-Tayyar, MD

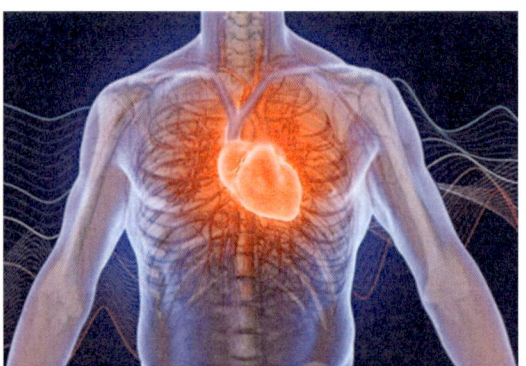

Case Study 1

A 23-year-old single lady presented to Family Medicine Clinic complaining of palpitation.

Doctor: Tell me more about your complain.
Patient Palpitation started in six months. It occurs daily, most of the time with no clear precipitating or relieving factors.

Doctor: What are the associated symptoms?
Patient: Insomnia and fatigue

Doctor: Do you consume caffeine?
Patient: Yes, a cup of Americano, 120 ml every morning, but this has been going on for the last three years.

On Examination:

Bp=130/67
P=110 B/M
General appearance: normal
CVS: S1+S2+0
Chest: clear
ECG: sinus tacky cardia

Labs:

Hb=12.5
Renal and hepatic profile and electrolytes are normal

Initial impression and plan:

- The initial diagnosis is over consumption of caffeine.
- Patient was advised to avoid caffeine totally and counseled about sleep hygiene.
- Came after three weeks, not improved at all.

Patient: I still feel my heart pump very quickly.

Doctor: As a review, you said you feel rapid heartbeats most of the time for the last six months, no obvious precipitating or reliving factors and associated with insomnia and fatigue, is that correct?

Patient: Yes.

Doctor: Anything you would like to add?

Patient: No.

Doctor: Do you have regular menstrual cycle? Have you noticed weight change?

Patient: I have regular menses, but yes, I lost 12 pounds though my appetite and eating habit are as usual.

Doctor: Do you have excessive sweating?

Patient: I have noticed that recently.

This time doctor added TSH.

TSH came as 0.001 mlunit/l (low).

Then FT4 and FT3 were requested urgently.

FT4 came as 70 pmol/l (11.5–22.7 pmol/L) and free T3 as 8 pmlo/l (3.5–6.5 pmol/L).

The most likely diagnosis is hyperthyroidism.

Case Discussion

This patient complained of palpitation for six months. No significant difference between resting & exertion so Anemia is unlikely. The amount of caffeine intake is not significant and the patient is consuming the same amount of caffeine even before the onset of the illness, this makes the diagnosis of caffeine overuse unlikely.

Energy drinks contain large amount of caffeine as well. Other substance that can cause palpitation including, tobacco, alcohol, amphetamine and cannabis. We should consider substance abuse among student and people with jobs require staying awake for long time (securities & trucks drivers).

Hyperthyroidism causes palpitation, associated with insomnia and fatigue. Also can cause muscle pain, menstrual irregularity, hair falling, nervousness, weight loss. It is not necessary to have all the manifestations at the same time. Some manifestations can give a clue about the diagnosis. These symptoms confusing with anxiety disorder and emotional stress. For that: evaluation of the psychological status of the patient as well as systemic review are very important.

Female hormonal changes related to pregnancy or menstrual cycle also sometimes are associated with palpitations but it is temporary and of no concern. Some acute conditions like fever, can cause palpitations. One Celsius degree elevation in the body temperature can cause a 10 beat/min increase in heartbeat. Dehydration and Electrolytes imbalance both can cause palpitations. So, patients with acute gastroenterology symptoms whether acute or chronic can develop palpitations.

References

1. Weber, B. and Kapoor, W., 1996. Evaluation and outcomes of patients with palpitations. The American Journal of Medicine, 100(2), pp.138-148.
2. JERI R, R. and Wheeler, S., 2005. Hyperthyroidism: Diagnosis and Treatment. Am Fam Physician, 15(72(4), pp.623-630.
3. KRAVETS, I., 2016. Hyperthyroidism: Diagnosis and Treatment. Am Fam Physician, 1(93(5), pp.363-370.

Case Study 2

A 26-year-old lady, single with regular menstrual cycle presented to Family Medicine Clinic complaining of palpitation for the last two months.

Doctor: Tell me more about your complain.
Patient: I have episodes of rapid heartbeats almost every day and for the last three days it awakes me up from sleep.

Doctor: Tell me more about your symptoms
Patient: I have this fast heart beat associated with shortness of breath and chest pain. I think I'm dying or losing my mind during the episode.

Doctor: What is the duration of each episode?
Patient: About 15 minutes.

Doctor: Is it associated with headache or dizziness?
Patient: Sometimes.

Doctor: What are the other associated symptoms rather than SOB?
Patient: Sweating, numbness and tremor.

Doctor: Did you experience a loss of consciousness during the episode?
Patient: No.

Doctor: Are you stressed recently?
Patient: Yes. I'm newly holding position of restaurant manager and I want to prove myself.

Doctor: Do you have a family history of any tumor or malignancies

Patient: No.

On Examination:

BMI=23
BP =123/82
P=70 b/m
CVS: S1+S2+0
ECG: normal

Labs:

CBC, Renal and Hepatic profiles are normal.
Thyroid function is normal.

Initial Diagnosis and plan:

- Initial diagnosis: Pheochromocytoma.
- Patient requested to do 24 hour urine collection for catecholamine's and metanephrines and the result came normal.
- Drug screening came also as normal, the patient came back to the doctor.

What is the most likely diagnosis?

Panic Attacks

Case Discussion

This lady is complaining of episodic palpitation, associated with SOB, chest pain, numbness and sweating, each episode stays for less than 30 minutes, peaks at 10 minutes then disappears by itself. It is characteristic of panic attacks.

Panic attacks are more common among young adults and among adolescents. Twice common in females. This patient has no symptoms suggested of hyperthyroidism in spite of that hyperthyroidism needs to be ruled out.

It might confuse also with Pheochromocytoma or temporal lobe epilepsy.

Pheochromocytoma is an uncommon, typically noncancerous (benign) tumor that emerges in the adrenal glands and is characterized by the release of catecholamines. These hormones, such as adrenaline and noradrenaline, can induce symptoms like high blood pressure, headaches, and excessive sweating.

While most pheochromocytomas are identified in individuals aged 20 to 50, the tumor can develop at any stage of life. Diagnosis often involves initial screening through a 24-hour urine collection to measure catecholamine levels, followed by imaging studies such as an adrenal MRI or MIBG scan to confirm the diagnosis definitively.

Palpitation in General

Elevated or irregular perception of the heartbeat, known as palpitations, is a frequent symptom among individuals seeking assistance from family physicians. While palpitations can indicate serious cardiac arrhythmias that pose a potential threat, the majority of cases are harmless. Palpitations may arise from various sources, including cardiac arrhythmias, non-arrhythmic cardiac factors, extracardiac origins, psychiatric factors, and medication-related causes.

Cardiac Arrhythmias

- Atrial fibrillation/flutter
- block or sinus node dysfunction
- Bradycardia-tachycardia syndrome (sick sinus syndrome)
- Multifocal atrial tachycardia
- Premature supraventricular or ventricular contractions
- Sinus tachycardia or arrhythmia
- Supraventricular tachycardia
- Ventricular tachycardia
- Wolff-Parkinson-White syndrome

References

1. Weber, B. and Kapoor, W., 1996. Evaluation and outcomes of patients with palpitations. The American Journal of Medicine, 100(2), pp.138-148.

2. HAM, P., WATERS, A. and OLIVER, M., 2003. Treatment of Panic Disorder. Am Fam Physician, 15(71(4), pp.733-739.

Case Study 3

A 14-year-old girl came to the family physician with generalized fatigue and palpitation for the last one month.

Doctor: What is your complaint?
Patient: I feel that I am tired, quickly fatigued and with minimal effort I feel my heart beat.

Doctor: When did this start?
Patient: I can't remember but at least one month.
Patient's mother: I noticed that her skin and lips are pale. She also is not performing well at school.

Doctor: Any other problems?
Patient mother: She had menarche last year and she has heavy menstruation.

Doctor: Any other bleeding?
Patient: No.

On Examination:
Vital signs: HR 105b/m, BP: 95/65 RR: 12b/m
Head and Neck exam: pale sclera and pale lips
Cardiovascular: S1 + S2 and systolic murmur
Abdomen: normal

Doctor: Okay, it is very likely that she has anemia. We will do a blood test and will see you next week.
Blood was done at 10 am, the result was back within one hour and the lab called the requesting physician for a critical result.

Lab: I have a critical result I want to notify.
Doctor: Yes.

Lab: Patient (name), has hemoglobin of 5.7g/dl.
Doctor: Thank you.

The doctor immediately asked the nurse to call the patient to come back to the hospital immediately.
Patient came to the Family Medicine Clinic from home.
Family medicine doctor called ER.

FM Doc: I have a patient with critically low Hemoglobin 5.7 and symptomatic with palpitation. I will send her immediately to the ER.
ER Doc: Okay.

In ER patient received and seen by ER physician and labs was as follow:
WBC normal
Hemoglobin 5.7
MCV 65
Plt 500
Other blood parameter was normal.
Viral signs was the same as in FM clinic.
The emergency ordered 2 units of pRBCs to be transfused.
After two hours the blood arrived and the first unit was transfused.
15 minutes into transfusion the patient started to develop rash and fever, blood was stopped.
Patient was kept and under observation so was admitted for one day under internal medicine.
Hematology was called on the second day when repeated Hb was 5.8.
Hematology advised IV iron immediately and arranged follow up in the clinic.

Corrected Scenario

Lab: I have a critical result I want to notify.
Doctor: Yes.

Lab: Patient (name), has hemoglobin of 5.7g/dl.
Doctor: Thank you.

The doctor called hematology.

FM doc: I have an urgent consultation.
Hematology: Okay.

FM Doc: I have a young lady who is vitally stable but had symptomatic iron deficiency anemia with Hb of 5.7.
Hematology: Okay, we will see her tomorrow in the infusion for IV iron or if there is no appointment we will ask patient to come to ER to receive the first IV iron dose.

Discussion

This case represents a girl with symptomatic iron deficiency anemia, most likely related to the heavy menstrual bleeding. The cause of heavy menstruation may need further evaluation along with review of patient's dietary habits.

Such cases of anemia usually present with symptoms but with no hemodynamic instability because the anemia is developing gradually and the affected person is young who can tolerate low levels of hemoglobin without hemodynamic instability.

In such scenario urgent action need to be taken but avoidance of blood product is best option for two reasons:

1. Patient is young and will tolerate anemia well especially when it is chronic.
2. In young females, the exposure to blood products will cause allo-antibodies which will have complications in future pregnancies.

The patient had developed a reaction to blood products which is likely a minor reaction that will resolve with stop of transfusion with no major complications.

In such a scenario IV iron is a better option as symptomatic patients on oral iron will take a long time to act.

It will be very useful to put her on oral iron after the IV iron until the cause of her disease discovered.

References

1. Peyrin-Biroulet, L., Williet, N. and Cacoub, P., 2015. Guidelines on the diagnosis and treatment of iron deficiency across indications: a systematic review. The American Journal of Clinical Nutrition, 102(6), pp.1585-1594.
2. Goddard, A., James, M., McIntyre, A. and Scott, B., 2011. Guidelines for the management of iron deficiency anemia. Gut, 60(10), pp.1309-1316.
3. Barish, C., Bregman, D., Butcher, A., Koch, T. and Morris, D., 2011. Safety and Efficacy of High Dose Intravenous Ferric Carboxymaltose vs. Standard Medical Care in the Treatment of Iron Deficiency Anemia. American Journal of Gastroenterology, 106, pp. S406-S407.

Case Study 4

A 24-year-old man presents to the clinic complaining of palpitations.

Physician: Since when did you notice the palpitation?
Patient: maybe three weeks.

Physician: Is there any chest pain?
Patient: No.

Physician: Do you have Bronchial Asthma?
Patient: No.

Physician: Did you notice neck swelling, weight loss or diarrhea?
Patient: No.

Physician: You are still young for heart diseases, we will do some labs to rule out Anemia or over active thyroid first then if normal you need psychiatry assessment for anxiety.

Case 4 Corrected
A 24-year-old man presents to the clinic complaining of palpitations.
Physician: since when did you notice the palpitation?

Patient: Maybe three weeks.
Physician: Is there any chest pain?

Patient: No.
Physician: Do you have Bronchial Asthma?

Patient: No.

Physician: Did you notice neck swelling, weight loss or diarrhea?

Patient: No.

Physician: Can you tell me more about the palpitation?

Patient: I am having difficulties sleeping as well.

During history, physician notices the patient is hyperactive.

On Examination:

On examination his temperature is 38.5, BP 150/90 Pulse 110 regular, but no neurologic deficits.

Physician calls patient's home and finds out that the patient is living with his mother after his father passed away 15 years ago. He did not do well in school and thus could not complete his primary education.

Physician further found out that he had difficulties staying in a job and is fired due to recurrent absence. Mom is concerned since he lately started staying longer times outside home and she noticed odd behaviors as well. She thinks he could be using recreational drugs.

After facing the patient with theses information's and clarifying the dangerous complications we must avoid he admits being using amphetamine tablets daily for the last months.

Junior Physician Mistakes:

- Physician jumped to conclusion without assessing the full picture
- Physician failed to examine the patient.
- Physician didn't explore the patients social and familial history

Pearls and Take-Home Massages

• In 2013, the National Survey of Drug Use and Health reported a methamphetamine usage prevalence of 4.7% among individuals aged 12 or older in the United States.

• Amphetamines exhibit two primary pharmacological actions, namely central nervous system (CNS) stimulation and sympathomimetic effects. Therefore, an assessment should investigate signs of these effects, ranging from mild agitation to pronounced hyperactivity or seizures. Such behavior might be accompanied by severe psychosis, including hallucinations and paranoid delusions.

• Clinical diagnosis of amphetamine toxicity relies on recognizing key features such as agitation, hyperthermia, tachycardia, hypertension, and excessive sweating.

References

1. Sarayu Vasan and Olango, G.J. (2019). Amphetamine Toxicity. [online] Nih.gov. Available at: https://www.ncbi.nlm.nih.gov/books/NBK470276/.
2. bestpractice.bmj.com. (n.d.). Amphetamine overdose – Symptoms, diagnosis and treatment | BMJ Best Practice US. [online] Available at: https://bestpractice.bmj.com/topics/en-us/341 [Accessed 4 May 2021].

Urinary Incontinence

Abdulaziz A. Alghamdi, MD
Abdulraheem M. Bayameen, MD

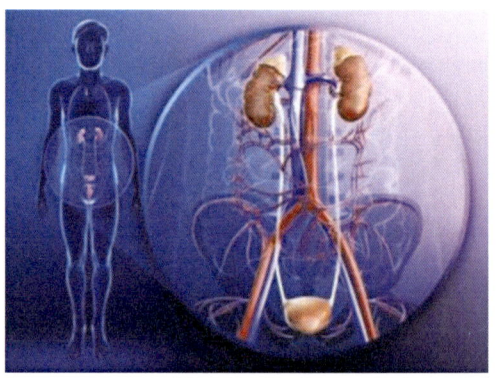

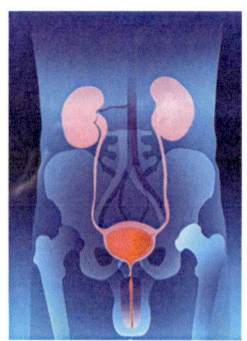

Case Study 1

This is a 35-year-old female known case of bronchial asthma presenting to the Family Medicine Clinic complaining of a urinary problem.

Physician: What kinds of urinary problem do you have?
Patient: I notice passing small amount of urine, I feel my pants wet during daytime.

Physician: Since how long?
Patient: Since many years but it increase in the last few months.

Physician: How much amount of leak?
Patient: The amount is little.

Physician: Is there anything that can precipitate this?
Patient: Yes it occurs when I have cough or abdominal strain.

Physician: Do you control yourself before going to the bathroom?
Patient: Yes.

Physician: Do you have dysuria?
Patient: No.

Physician: How is your symptoms of asthma?
Patient: I still have cough and SOB daily, although I take my only medication, which is Ventolin inhaler.

Physician: It seems we need to review your technique of using inhalers and adding another daily inhaler which can improve your symptoms.

Junior Clinic Physician Mistakes:

- Physician didn't take his time to think more about the differential diagnosis.
- Searching for fast fixed diagnosis.
- Physician managed the precipitating factor which is poorly controlled bronchial asthma but forgot to manage the main cause which is urinary incontinence.

Correct Scenario

This is a 35-year-old female known case of bronchial asthma presenting to the Family Medicine Clinic complaining of a urinary problem.

Physician: What kinds of urinary problem do you have?
Patient: I notice passing small amount of urine, I feel my pants wet during daytime.

Physician: Since how long?
Patient: Since many years but it increased in the last few months.

Physician: How much amount of leak?
Patient: The amount is little.

Physician: Is there anything that can precipitate this?
Patient: Yes it's occur when I have cough or abdominal strain.

Physician: Do you control yourself before going to the bathroom?
Patient: Yes.

Physician: Do you have dysuria?
Patient: No.

Physician: Are you married?
Patient: Yes.

Physician: How many kids do you have? And are all of them had normal deliveries?

Patient: I have eight kids and all of them are spontaneous vaginal deliveries except the last one it was Caesarean.

Physician: Regarding your menstrual cycle, is it regular?
Patient: Yes.

Physician: How is your symptoms of asthma?
Patient: I still have cough and SOB daily although I take my only medication, which is Ventolin inhaler.

Physician: It seems we need to review your technique of using inhalers and adding another daily inhaler which can improve your symptoms.

Physician asks for urine analysis and culture, renal function test and renal ultra sound.

Physician diagnosed her as stress incontinence due to multiparous and weak pelvic floor muscles after he did all the investigations, which was unremarkable, and referred her to OBG. Also he referred her to the health educator to review her technique of using the inhaler.

Case Discussion

Urinary incontinence, the involuntary loss of urine, includes stress incontinence triggered by physical activities like coughing, laughing, sneezing, running, or lifting, exerting pressure on the bladder and causing leakage. It's important to clarify that stress incontinence is not linked to psychological stress.

Several factors heighten the risk of urinary incontinence:

1. Pregnancy and vaginal childbirth
2. Obesity
3. A family history of incontinence
4. Aging, although incontinence isn't an unavoidable aspect of getting older

5. Non-surgical treatments

Initially, a general practitioner may suggest simple measures to assess symptom improvement, such as:

1. Adopting lifestyle changes, including weight loss and reducing caffeine and alcohol intake.
2. Performing pelvic floor exercises to strengthen muscles through contractions.
3. Undergoing bladder training to learn techniques for delaying the urge to urinate.
4. Using incontinence products like absorbent pads and handheld urinals.
5. Considering medication if symptoms persist despite other measures.

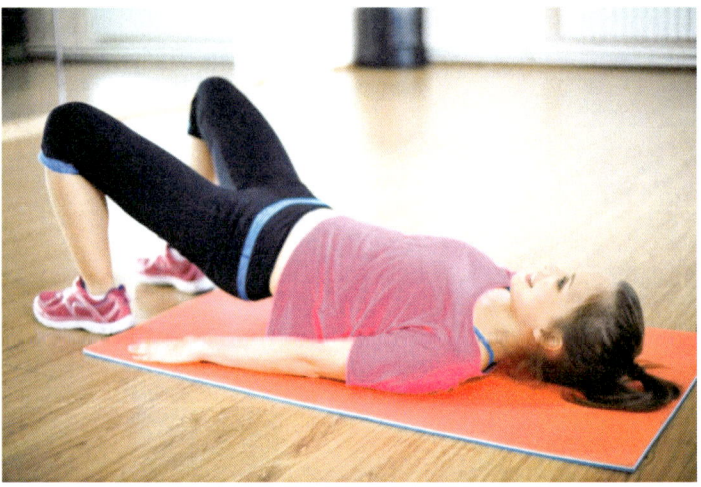

Figure 17: showing Pelvic floor exercises

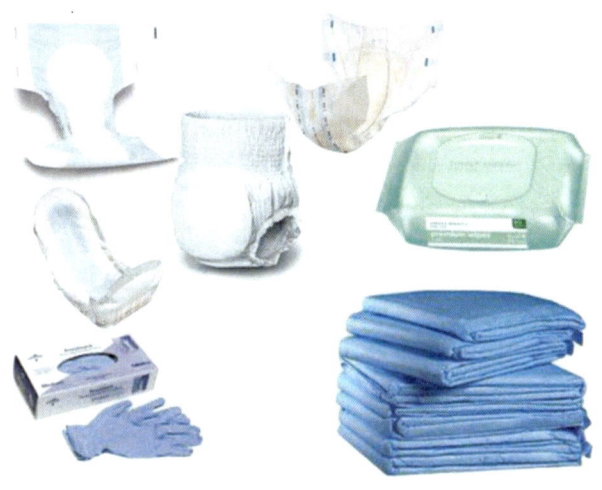

Figure 18: showing Incontinence products

References

1. NHS Choices (2019). Overview – Urinary incontinence. [online] NHS. Available at: https://www.nhs.uk/conditions/urinary-incontinence/.
2. Mayo Clinic. (n.d.). Stress incontinence – Symptoms and causes. [online] Available at: https://www.mayoclinic.org/diseases-conditions/stress-incontinence/symptoms-causes/syc-20355727#:~:text=Urinary%20incontinence%20is%20the%20unintentional%20loss%20of%20urine.
3. BetterPT Blog. (2019). What to Know About the Pelvic Floor and Exercises Postpartum. [online] Available at: https://www.betterpt.com/post/what-to-know-about-the-pelvic-floor-and-exercises-postpartum.
4. www.facebook.com. (n.d.). Colin DME – Colin DME updated their cover photo. [online] Available at: https://www.facebook.com/colindmergv/photos/pb.111423260381886.-2207520000./118090913048454/.

Case Study 2

A 70-year-old male known case of HTN, coming from a rural area, not seeking any medical advice for many years. He came to the Family Medicine Clinic complaining of urinary problems.

Physician: What kind of urinary problem do you have?
Patient: I pass large amounts of urine without feeling all the time of the day.

Physician: For how long is this issue with you?
Patient: For few months.

Physician: As you said, it's happening most of the day, but is there anything that makes this more frequent?
Patient: Yes, when I cough or sneeze.

Physician: Can you control yourself before going to the toilet?
Patient: No.

Physician: Do you feel pain when you pass the urine?
Patient: Yes, it hurts like burning sensation.

Physician: Are you taking any medications?
Patient: I take this medication for HTN (Amlodipine).

On Examination:

- V\S stable.
- Abdomen: unremarkable

- PR: large smooth prostate.

Physician orders urine analysis and culture which returns normal, and he requests some blood works which is also normal.

Physician diagnosed him as early presentation of BPH and started him on medications.

Junior Physician Mistakes:

- Physician did not take full detail history of the patients complains.
- This is not a typical early presentation of BPH esp. for patient's coming from a rural area and not seeking any medical advice before.
- Physician thinks this is a simple BPH as the patient is old age and has findings in the examination but he didn't utilize his tools like ordering an ultrasound.
- This scenario is compatible to complicated or neglected BPH which causes a decompensated urinary bladder with overflow urinary incontinence and presented with potential retention.

Correct Scenario

A 70-year-old male known case of HTN, coming from a rural area, not seeking any medical advice for many years. He came to the Family Medicine Clinic complaining of urinary problems.

Physician: What kind of urinary problem do you have?
Patient: I pass large amounts of urine without feeling all the time of the day.

Physician: For how long is this issue with you?
Patient: For few months.

Physician: As you said, it happens most of the day, but is there anything that makes this more frequent?
Patient: Yes when I cough or sneeze.

Physician: Can you control yourself before going to the toilet?
Patient: No.

Physician: Do you feel pain when you pass the urine?
Patient: Yes, it hurts like burning sensation.
Physician: Is this burning sensation new onset?
Patient: No, I have this for many years but I didn't seek any medical advice.

Physician: How many times do you go to the toilet?
Patient: I go to the toilet after I wet myself without feeling.

Physician: What other symptoms do you notice when you go to the toilet?
Patient: I take time to start urination and at the end it ends with drops, all of this was for a long time.

Physician: Are you taking any medications?
Patient: I take this medication for HTN (Amlodipine).

On Examination:

- V\S stable.
- Abdomen: unremarkable
- PR: large smooth prostate.

Physician orders urine analysis and culture which returns normal, and he requests some blood works which is also normal.

In addition, he requests an ultrasound which shows a huge urinary bladder volume more than 500cc post void. Prostate was big with hydroureteronephrosis.

He diagnosed the patient as decompensated urinary bladder secondary to long standing BPH with potential urinary retention.

He orders a folly's catheter insertion, BPH medications and referred him to urology clinic.

Case Discussion

1. Obstructive uropathy is a common condition characterized by a disruption in normal urinary flow, resulting from either anatomical or functional issues. This problem tends to become more prevalent

with age, often being associated with conditions such as benign prostatic hyperplasia or neurogenic bladder.
2. When the regular flow of urine through the urinary tract is hindered, it causes a backup of urine into the kidney's collecting system. Over time, this backup can lead to dilation within the tract, and the development of obstructive nephropathy occurs as the kidney's filtration system is impacted. The mechanism involves various factors, including local ischemia due to distention and increased intratubular pressures. In cases of partial obstruction, there is an upregulation of angiotensin and AT1-receptor, promoting increased ureteral peristalsis to alleviate the obstruction.
3. The approach to treating obstructive uropathy focuses on promptly addressing the obstructive problem. Therapies are guided by bladder volume measurements, and an initial step may involve attempting a Foley catheter, typically using a 16 or 18-Fr Foley, especially if the obstruction is attributed to common causes like benign prostatic hypertrophy or hyperplasia.

References

1. Tseng, T.Y. and Stoller, M.L. (2009). Obstructive uropathy. Clinics in Geriatric Medicine, [online] 25(3), pp.437–443. Available at: https://pubmed.ncbi.nlm.nih.gov/19765491/.
2. Rishor-Olney, C.R. and Hinson, M.R. (2020). Obstructive Uropathy. [online] PubMed. Available at: https://www.ncbi.nlm.nih.gov/books/NBK558921/.
3. National Institute on Aging. (n.d.). Urinary Incontinence in Older Adults. [online] Available at: https://www.nia.nih.gov/health/urinary-incontinence-older-adults#:~:text=Urinary%20incontinence%20means%20a%20person.

Case Study 3

A 50-yearsold female known case of DM. She came to the Family Medicine Clinic and complained of urinary problems.

Physician: What kind of urinary problems do you have?
Patient: I start to pass urine before I reach the toilet.

Physician: For how long is this issue with you?
Patient: This issue started one year ago.

Physician: Did this problem happen to you before one year?
Patient: Actually, it started seven7 years ago but it was very mild and only when I cough but in this year it increased and I pass urine before I reach the toilet.

Physician: Do you still pass urine when you cough?
Patient: Yes.

Physician: Do you feel pain when you pass the urine?
Patient: Yes, it hurt like burning sensation.

Physician: How many times you go to toilet?
Patient: I go a lot.

Physician: How many kids do you have?
Patient: I have seven.

Physician: How old the youngest one?
Patient: Seven years old.

On Examination:

- V\S stable.
- Positive cough stress test.

Physician orders urine analysis which is normal and culture (mixed growth).
Physician also orders Ultrasound urinary tract which shows Prevoid 200cc and postvoid 0cc.
Physician diagnosed her as stress incontinence.
Physician starts her on antibiotics and refers her to OBG.

Junior Physician Mistake:

- Physician did not think of other possible causes of the patient complain.
- Physician didn't take any history of the chronic illness of the patient which is diabetes
- This patient has poorly controlled diabetes for many years which caused her bladder to be overactive and she needs in addition to the management done by the physician to control her diabetes and to be started on anticholinergic medication.
- This scenario is compatible to mixed urinary incontinence: stress incontinence due to weak pelvic floor due to multiparous and Urge incontinence due to overactive urinary bladder due to poor controlled DM.

Correct Scenario

A 50-yearold female known case of DM. She come to the Family Medicine Clinic complain of urinary problems.

Physician: What kind of urinary problems do you have?
Patient: I start to pass urine before I reach the toilet.

Physician: For how long is this issue with you?
Patient: This issue started one year ago.

Physician: Did this problem happen to you before one year?

Patient: Actually, it started 7 years ago but it was very mild and only when I cough but in this year it increased and I pass urine before I reach the toilet.

Physician: Do you still pass urine when you cough?

Patient: Yes.

Physician: Do you feel pain when you pass the urine?

Patient: Yes, it is hurt like burning sensation.

Physician: How many times you go to toilet?

Patient: I go a lot.

Physician: How many kids do you have?

Patient: I have seven.

Physician: How old the youngest one?

Patient: Seven years old.

Physician: What medications you are taking right now?

Patient: I am taking my diabetic medications.

Physician: Let's talk about your diabetes, what's your usual blood sugar readings?

Patient: It's usually high, more than 350 mg/dl despite using my medications.

Physician: Your last HbA1c between 12-14 over the last few years, we need to take actions to bring it down, I will change or add some medications if you agree with me?

Patient: Sure.

On Examination:

- V\S stable.
- Positive cough stress test.

Physician orders urine analysis which is normal and culture (mixed growth)

Physician also orders Ultrasound urinary tract which shows Prevoid 200cc and postvoid 0cc.

Physician diagnosed her as mixed urinary incontinence: stress incontinence due to weak pelvic floor due to multiparous and Urge incontinence due to overactive urinary bladder due to poorly controlled DM.

Physician starts her on antibiotics, changes her DM medications and refers her to OBG and Urology services.

Clinical Pearls and Take-Home Messages

Mixed Urinary Incontinence is the involuntary leakage associated with Stress Urinary Incontinence and Urge Urinary Incontinence and can also include Nocturia and dribbling. Some people have a mixture of all these different symptoms which may have several different causes.

References

1. Bladder & Bowel Community. (2017). Mixed Urinary Incontinence. [online] Available at: https://www.bladderandbowel.org/bladder/bladder-conditions-and-symptoms/mixed-urinary-incontinence/#:~:text=Mixed%20Urinary%20Incontinence%20is%20the.
2. Gomelsky, A. and Dmochowski, R.R. (2011). Treatment of mixed urinary incontinence. Central European Journal of Urology, 64, pp.120–126.
3. Healthline. (2017). Mixed Incontinence: What is It and How Can You Treat It? [online] Available at: https://www.healthline.com/health/overactive-bladder/mixed-incontinence#treatment [Accessed 6 Feb. 2022].

Case Study 4

A 55-year-old male came to the Family Medicine Clinic complaining of urinary problems, his last visit to the clinic was two years ago.

Physician: What is your complain today?
Patient: Sometimes I wet my pants before reaching the bathroom if I went late.

Physician: For how long do you have this problem?
Patient: Since few months.

Physician: What other urinary symptoms do you have?
Patient: I feel dribbling at the end of urination and incomplete voiding sensation, so I go again to the bathroom especially at night, which interferes with my sleep.

Physician: Do you have any other symptoms like fever, flank pain, blood in the urine?
Patient: No other symptoms.

Physician: Did you take any medications for that?
Patient: No.

Physician: Do have any chronic medical illnesses like diabetes, hypertension?
Patient: No, I did investigations 2 years ago and it was normal.

Physician: Did you undergo any operations before?
Patient: Only appendectomy 30 years ago.

Physician: Did you take any medications, or seek any medical advice?

Patient: No, but I remember my elder brother had same symptoms and diagnosed as an enlarge prostate.

On Examination:

- V\S stable.
- PR: shows an enlarged prostate.

Physician ordered a urine culture, which showed no growth and normal renal function.

He thinks the patient has BPH and orders an ultrasound which showed no hydronephrosis only bilateral fullness of renal pelvis and normal wall thickening of urinary bladder with the pre-void 400 mL and post void 45 mL and prostate 50 g.

So BPH medication has prescribed for the patient.

Junior Physician Mistake:

- Physician did not analyze the chief complaint of the patient like the amount of urine, urine flow, and dysuria.
- Physician did not ask about the family history of diabetes or diuretic medications use.
- He did not check the urine for glucose and random blood sugar.
- A physician depended on the last visit investigation two years ago.

Correct Scenario

A 55-year-old male come to the Family Medicine Clinic complaining of urinary problems, his last visit to the clinic was two years ago.

Physician: What is your complaint today?

Patient: I got to the bathroom too much especially at night which interferes with my sleep sometimes I wet my pants before reaching the bathroom if I went late.

Physician: For how long do you have this problem?
Patient: Since few months.
Physician: Did you take any medications for that?
Patient: No.

Physician: What other urinary symptoms do you have?
Patient: I feel dribbling at the end of urination and incomplete voiding sensation so I go again to the bathroom.

Physician: What about the amount and flow of urine?
Patient: It's a very large amount with intermittent flow but not always.

Physician: Do you have any other symptoms like fever, flank pain, blood in the urine?
Patient: No other symptoms.

Physician: Do have any chronic medical illnesses like diabetes, hypertension?
Patient: No, I did investigations two years ago and it was normal.

Physician: Do you have a family history of diabetes or other diseases?
Patient: Yes my parents and elder sister have diabetes.

Physician: Did you do any operations before?
Patient: Only appendectomy 30 years ago.

Physician: Did you do take any medication, or sought any medical advice?
Patient: No, but I remember my elder brother has same symptoms and diagnosed as an enlarge prostate.

On Examination:

- V\S stable.
- PR: shows an enlarged prostate.

Physician orders a urine analysis which shows glucose 4 plus (high) without leukocyte in urine and negative nitrate.

So he order RBS which was 450 mg/dl.

Then the physician orders a renal function test, hemoglobin A1c with lipid profile.

Renal function test comes normal hemoglobin A1c: 9 and the lipid profile was high.

Also he ordered an ultrasound & KUB which showed no hydronephrosis only bilateral fullness of the renal pelvis and normal wall thickening of the urinary bladder with the pre-void 400 mL and post void 45 mL and prostate 50 g most.

So he diagnosed him as newly diagnosed diabetes and dyslipidemia plus BPH.

Patient has early urinary symptom of BPH associated with polyuria secondary to diuretic effect of uncontrolled newly diabetes (Urge because of diabetes and transient incontinence as a complication of DM).

Clinical Pearls and Take-Home Messages

Type 2 diabetes, impacting 90%–95% of individuals with diabetes, has been linked to bladder dysfunction, particularly affecting the detrusor muscle. The impaired detrusor function results in a diminished maximum flow rate given a specific level of bladder outlet resistance, leading to increased post-void residual and more severe lower urinary tract symptoms (LUTS). Benign prostatic hyperplasia (BPH) also manifests with LUTS, featuring reduced maximum urinary flow rate and heightened post-void residual.

Despite the shared symptomatology, the underlying pathophysiology differs. BPH primarily enhances bladder outlet resistance through static and dynamic components without directly impairing detrusor function.

Several mechanisms elucidate how diabetes may influence BPH. Firstly, changes in insulin concentrations may impact sex hormone levels, sympathetic nerve activity, and/or the insulin-like growth factor axis, influencing prostate growth. Moreover, poorly controlled diabetes, through osmotic diuresis, can contribute to urinary frequency and nocturia, affecting LUTS via neuropathic mechanisms that influence both motor and sensory nerves.

References

1. Sarma, A.V., St. Sauver, J.L., Hollingsworth, J.M., Jacobson, D.J., McGree, M.E., Dunn, R.L., Lieber, M.M. and Jacobsen, S.J. (2012). Diabetes Treatment and Progression of Benign Prostatic Hyperplasia in Community-dwelling Black and White Men. Urology, 79(1), pp.102–108.
2. Sarma, A.V., Burke, J.P., Jacobson, D.J., McGree, M.E., St. Sauver, J., Girman, C.J., Lieber, M.M., Herman, W., Macoska, J., Montie, J.E. and Jacobsen, S.J. (2007). Associations between Diabetes and Clinical Markers of Benign Prostatic Hyperplasia Among Community-Dwelling Black and White Men. Diabetes Care, 31(3), pp.476–482.
3. Diabetes in Control (2006). Diabetes Tied to Enlarged Prostate. [online] Diabetes in Control. A free weekly diabetes newsletter for Medical Professionals. Available at: https://www.diabetesincontrol.com/diabetes-tied-to-enlarged-prostate/ [Accessed 6 Feb. 2022].
4. IDDT. (n.d.). The Prostate and Diabetes. [online] Available at: https://www.iddt.org/related-health-issues/the-prostate-and-diabetes [Accessed 6 Feb. 2022].

Dyspnea Chapter

Basmah O. Bamashmous, MD
Riham K. Elsayed, MD
Yusuf H. Vali, MD

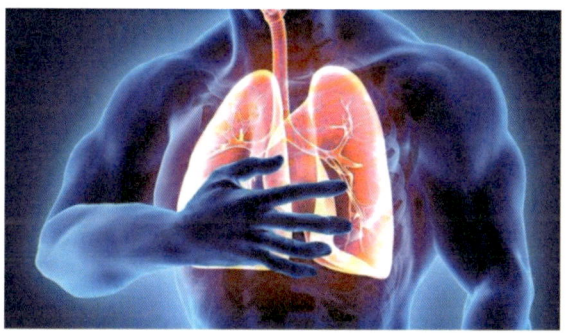

Case Study 1

A 17-year-old male patient known to have mild asthma since childhood presented with breathlessness. He had run out of his salbutamol inhaler one month previously.

Auscultation of his chest showed bilateral wheeze. He was therefore diagnosed with an asthma exacerbation and provided with a new supply of his salbutamol inhaler.

Q1) What are the important clinical features in the history of a patient with asthma which will help identify those patients at an increased risk of adverse outcomes?

A1) There are a number of risk factors which are associated with poor outcomes and they should be sought for in the history. They include previous ICU admission, hospital admission within the last 12 months, poor adherence to treatment, frequent use of salbutamol, comorbidities such as depression, obesity, and also lack of an asthma self-management plan.

Q2) What are the important clinical findings which should be elicited when examining a patient with asthma?

A1) Peak expiratory flow rate, oxygen saturations, pulse rate, heart rate, respiratory rate, use of accessory muscles and ability to speak in full sentences.

These features will help assess the severity of the exacerbation and guide management.

Q3) What is the correct management plan in this situation?

The severity of the exacerbation and presence of risk factors for an adverse outcome will guide the acute and chronic management. There should be a very low threshold for prescribing a short course of high dose oral corticosteroids for patients with an asthma exacerbation. Equally important is to identify the reason for the presentation. Often it is due to poor control and this must be addressed to prevent future exacerbations and poor outcomes.

Salbutamol alone should never be used for asthma. In 2019 GINA made the most dramatic change to the asthma guidelines removing salbutamol (SABA) from step 1 of the asthma treatment strategy. All patients should have inhaled steroids (ICS). The preferred choice for patients with mild intermittent asthma on Step 1 or 2 of the treatment ladder is PRN ICS-formoterol combination such as symbicort. It is vital that inhaler technique is demonstrated and checked. A self-management plan should also be devised.

Patients with apparently mild asthma are at risk of serious adverse events (Dusser, Allergy 2007) 15–20% of adults dying of asthma had symptoms less than weekly in previous 3 months according to this study. Dispensing of ≥12 canisters of salbutamol per year is associated with higher risk of death (Suissa, AJRCCM 1994). It is therefore important to shift away from the practice of using PRN salbutamol for mild asthma. All patients should be educated on the use of inhaled steroids with an emphasis on correct inhaler technique which should be checked at every visit. For patients using ICS via a pressurized metered dose inhaler (MDI), they should take it using a spacer device. Patients should also be asked to gargle their throat after use of ICS to reduce the risk of oral candidiasis.

Reference

A Pocket Guide for Health Professionals Updated 2021 BASED ON THE GLOBAL STRATEGY FOR ASTHMA MANAGEMENT AND PREVENTION POCKET GUIDE FOR ASTHMA MANAGEMENT AND PREVENTION (for Adults and Children Older than 5 Years) (for Adults and Children Older than 5 Years) POCKET GUIDE FOR ASTHMA MANAGEMENT AND PREVENTION (for Adults and Children Older than 5 Years). (n.d.). [online] Available at: https://ginasthma.org/wp-content/uploads/2021/05/GINA-Pocket-Guide-2021-V2-WMS.pdf.

Case Study 2

A 66-year-old male known case of DM type 2, hypertension and dyslipidemia on regular follow up and medications.

He came to Family Medicine Clinic today complaining from shortening of breath, epigastric pain and abdominal pain which started suddenly today three hours ago.

On Examination:

He is alert and oriented to time and place.
Blood pressure is 170/90.
Respiratory rate is 20 b/m.
Pulse is 100 b/m.
O2 saturation is 99% upon breathing room air.

Physician: When did you notice the pain?
Patient: This morning. It is severe pain in my abdomen.

Physician: On a scale of 0 to 10 (In which 0 is no pain and 10 is the most severe pain you ever experienced) how severe is your pain?
Patient: 8.

Physician: What about your shortening of breath? When do you feel it and what increases it?
Patient: The shortness of breath started today with the abdominal pain and I even feel it even when I am at rest without any effort.

Physician: Did you notice any nausea, diarrhea or constipation?
Patient: I only noticed nausea.

Physician: Did you notice fever or any other respiratory problems?
Patient: No.

On Examination:

Abdomen was lax with mild tenderness on the epigastric region. No organomegaly noticed.

The Initial impression and plan:

The physician diagnosed the patient as gastritis and discharge him on PPI medication.

What went wrong in this consultation?

Incomplete history and physical examination lead to patient misdiagnosis and mismanagement.

Ideal Scenario

Physician: How do you feel your pain?
Patient: Severe pain in my abdomen.

Physician: On a scale of 0 to 10 how severe is your pain?
Patient: 8.

Physician: What about your shortening of breath when did you notice it? And what increases it?
Patient: it started with the abdominal pain today and I feel it even with rest without effort.

Physician: Is your pain referred to any other side?
Patient: I have some pain also radiating to my left shoulder.

Physicians: Are you taking your medication regularly?
Patient: Sometimes I forget some of them upon traveling.

Physician: Do you have any other respiratory or gastric symptoms?
Patient: No.

Physician: Are you a smoker?
Patient: Yes.

At the end of the Consultation, the physician talks to the patient:
I will do some investigation and order an ECG for you, and then I will see you again after the result.
So, the doctor here orders an ECG.

ECG Findings

- ST segment elevation in the anterior precordial leads.
- V1-V4: Anteroseptal injury.
- V3-V4: Anterior injury.
- V3-V6: Anterolateral injury. Leads I and aVL may also be involved, especially if the circumflex artery is affected (high lateral injury).
- Reciprocal ST segment depressions are often present in the inferior leads (II, III, aVF).

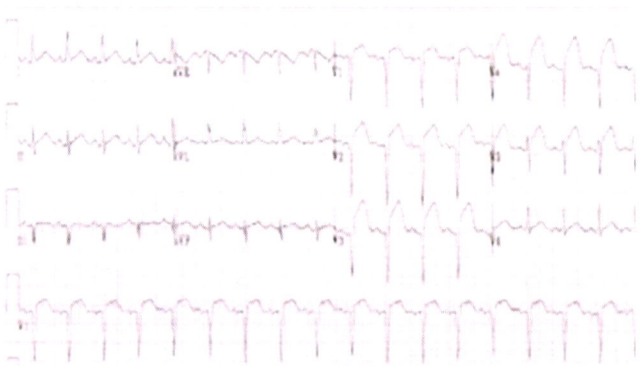

Figure 19: showing ECG Changes reflecting anterior MI

And the lab shows elevated **HS troponin level**.
The patient was diagnosed as a case of **ACUTE MI IN DM**.
He was referred urgently to cardiology for timely management.

Clinical Pearls and Take-Home Messages

- Myocardial infarction (MI) is a common cause of mortality in people with diabetes.
- IF any DM patient complaining of epigastric pain sever and sudden in nature, consider Silent MI and perform an urgent ECG.
- The case fatality from MI is high and may be reduced by thrombolysis, aspirin, beta-blockers and angiotensin-converting enzyme inhibitors.
- Poor metabolic control is common among diabetic patients with MI, and the importance of controlling blood glucose during and following an MI is paramount.
- Treatment with statins reduces cardiovascular mortality and morbidity in diabetic patients with previous MI (secondary prevention).
- Large studies in diabetic patients without existing heart disease have shown statistically insignificant reductions in cardiovascular emergencies as MI with improved glycemic control of the diabetes (primary prevention).
- Treating hypertension in people with diabetes prevents cardiovascular Morbidity and mortality.

References

1. Fisher, M. (1999). Diabetes and myocardial infarction. Best Practice & Research Clinical Endocrinology & Metabolism, 13(2), pp.331–343.
2. Cui, J., Liu, Y., Li, Y., Xu, F. and Liu, Y. (2021). Type 2 Diabetes and Myocardial Infarction: Recent Clinical Evidence and Perspective. Frontiers in Cardiovascular Medicine, 8.

Case Study 3

Ten-year-old boy, medically free, came to the Family Medicine Clinic complaining from shortness of breath, abdominal pain, nausea, vomiting two times today, fatigue, and frequent urination. He was at his friend's birthday party yesterday.

Physician: Since when he has these symptoms?
Patient's mother: From today morning.

Physician: Does he have a fever or diarrhea?
Patient's mother: No.

Physician: Does he have a cough or any respiratory symptoms?
Patient's mother: No.

Physician: Does he have burning micturition or loin pain?
Patient's mother: No.

Physician: Did he eat any food from outside?
Patient's mother: Yes, he was at his friend's birthday party yesterday and ate a lot of sweets and chocolates with cakes.

On Examination:

- Temperature: 36.5
- Respiratory rate: 20 b/m
- Heart rate: 98 b/m
- Blood pressure: 100/70

Patient is oriented to time, place, and person. Vitally stable.
Chest: free.
Abdomen: lax, moderate epigastric pain.
The physician diagnosed the patient as gastritis.

The physician reassured the patient's mother and discharged him the following:

- Domperidone Tablet (upon need).
- Stool analysis.
- Dietary advice and encouraged him to increase his water intake.

Ideal Scenario

Physician: Since when he has these symptoms?
Patient's mother: From today morning.

Physician: Is there recurrence of these symptoms?
Patient's mother: No.

Physician: Does he have fever or diarrhea?
Patient's mother: No.

Physician: Does he have cough or any respiratory symptoms?
Patient's mother: No.

Physician: Does he have burning micturition or loin pain?
Patient's mother: No.

Physician: Did he eat any food from outside?
Patient's mother: Yes, he was at his friend's birthday party yesterday and ate a lot of sweets and chocolates with cakes.

Physician: Is there a family history of diabetes mellitus?
Patient's mother: Yes, his father and grandfather are both diabetics.

On Examination:

- Temperature: 36.5
- Respiratory rate: 20 b/m
- Heart rate: 98 blm
- Blood pressure: 100/70

Patient is oriented to time, place and person. Vitally stable, has acetone (fruity) odor of breath.
Chest: free.
Abdomen: lax, moderate epigastric pain.
The physician orders some investigation to take the right decision.
(UDS, CBC, RBS, Anion gap, bicarbonate, chloride, blood PH, sodium, potassium and Renal function test.

*Result is like the following picture:

Glucose (mg/dl)	191
Arterial pH	7,04
Bicarbonate (mEq/l)	<3
Sodium (mEq/l)	136
Potassium (mEq/l)	4,8
Anion gap (mEq/l)	18
Serum and urine ketones	Positives
Creatinine (mg/dl)	0,77

Table 9: showing Lab results of the Case study

*Physician diagnosed patient as DKA.

- Start IV. Nacl 0.9% (sodium chloride solution)
- Urgent referral to ER Department for management.

Physician Mistakes:

- Did not take a complete history.
- Did not do complete physical examination.
- Did not cover all differential diagnosis of dyspnea with abdominal pain.
- Did not order the required laboratory examination.

Clinical Pearls and Take-Home Messages

- Family physician should screen for dyspnea red flags and differential diagnosis which include:
- Upper airway obstruction, metabolic acidosis (like DKA), acute cardiac problems (like MI), psychogenic disorder, bronchial asthma attacks, COPD, tension pneumothorax, congestive heart failure, pericardial tamponade, pulmonary embolism, interstitial lung disease, pneumonia & neuromuscular conditions.
- Diabetic ketoacidosis (DKA) is a common cause of hospital admission, morbidity, & mortality in children with T1DM.
- Diabetic ketoacidosis (DKA) is a common & recurrent problem for children with T1DM, due to lack of compliance on treatment & healthy lifestyle.
- Any patient (especially children), comes to you complaining from dyspnea & abdominal pain, with history of eating large amount of carbohydrates (especially if has positive family history for diabetes mellitus), you should examine for T1DM, & DKA.
- Lowering (HBA1c) has been associated with a reduction of microvascular & neuropathic complications of diabetes. In addition, it may lower the risk of myocardial infarction & cardiovascular death (ADA, Standards of Medical Care for Patients with Diabetes Mellitus).

References

1. Levitsky L. Death from diabetes (DM) in hospitalized children (1970-1988). Pediatr Res 1991; 29:A195.

2. Edge JA, Ford-Adams ME, Dunger DB. Causes of death in children with insulin dependent diabetes 1990-96. Arch Dis Child 1999; 81:318.
3. Curtis JR, To T, Muirhead S, et al. Recent trends in hospitalization for diabetic ketoacidosis in ontariochildren. Diabetes Care 2002; 25:1591.
4. Benoit SR, Zhang Y, Geiss LS, et al. Trends in Diabetic Ketoacidosis Hospitalizations and In-Hospital Mortality – United States, 2000-2014. MMWR Morb Mortal Wkly Rep 2018; 67:362.

Case Study 4

A 16-year-old boy, medically free came to the clinic with history of shortening of breath and chest pain today after he got hit by the ball during a football game last evening.

Vitals: was stable with O2 98% upon breathing room air and RR 18 b/m pulse 90 b/m.

Physician: Since when you have this shortening of breath and chest pain?
Patient: Only for two hours.

Physician: Do you have any cough or sputum?
Patient: No.

Physician: Can you describe this pain?
Patient: It started after I was hit by the ball in my Back below the right shoulder.

Physician: are you a smoker?
Patient: No, I am not.

Then, the physician starts to examine the patient and he explores his chest from the back, he sees the side of the ball trauma is reddish and tender.

After that physician diagnosed him as a chest wall trauma and gave him local and systemic analgesia.

Ideal Scenario

Physician: Since when you have this shortening of breath and chest pain?

Patient: Only for two hours.

Physician: Do you have any cough or sputum?

Patient: No.

Physician: Can you describe this pain?

Patient: It started after I was hit by the ball in my Back below the right shoulder.

Physician: what about the shortening of the breath do you have bronchial asthma?

Patient: No, I am not a bronchial asthma patient, and I did not take any medication for shortening of breath.

Physician: Are you smoker?

Patient: No, I am not.

The physician observes in that the patient is tall and thin, his height was 175cm and his weight was 50 kg.

So, physician does examination to the chest examination was normal with bronchial breathing in the left lung. But the right lung had unequal breath sounds, hyperresonance with percussion over the chest wall and decreased wall movement. Back examination: he has mild ecomosis at the site of the ball's trauma.

ECG was normal.

Chest x-ray Showed **RT pneumothorax.**

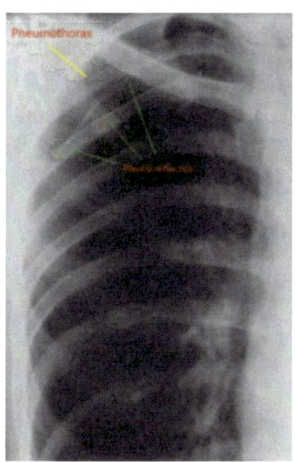

Figure 20: Chext x-ray showing rt Pnemothorax (green arrow)

Patient was sent to the Surgery Department to proceed for underwater seal chest tube insertion.

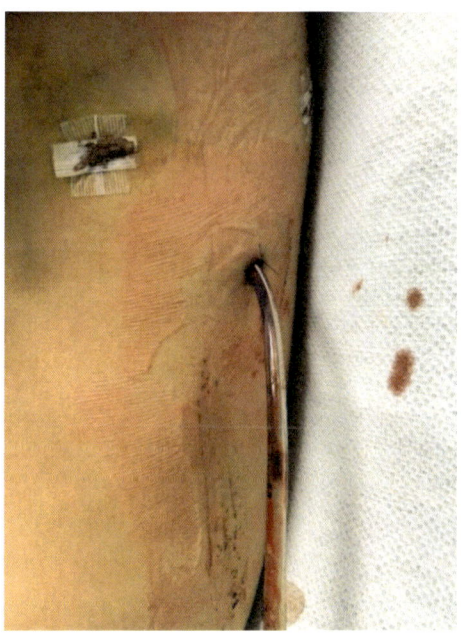

Figure 21: showing Underwater seal chest tube

Take-Home Message

- Ensuring safety as a physician entail conducting a thorough examination and refraining from hastily settling on the initial diagnosis.

A doctor's proficiency includes sharp observational skills.

Ordering an ECG is a crucial step for any patient presenting with acute chest pain.

- Primary spontaneous pneumothorax occurs in individuals without known respiratory conditions, often in the younger age group, whereas secondary spontaneous pneumothorax occurs in those with pre-existing pulmonary diseases.
- Tension pneumothorax demands immediate decompression, constituting a medical emergency.
- Patients with pneumothorax typically manifest dyspnea and chest pain.
- In tension pneumothorax, distress is evident through rapid, labored breathing, cyanosis, profuse sweating, and tachycardia.
- Initial treatment for pneumothorax is determined by clinical features, size/type of pneumothorax, and may involve observation with supplemental oxygen, percutaneous aspiration, chest drain insertion, and, in specific cases, video-assisted thoracoscopy (VATS) or thoracostomy.
- Individuals experiencing spontaneous pneumothoraxes face an elevated risk of recurrence.

References

1. bestpractice.bmj.com. (n.d.). Pneumothorax – Symptoms, diagnosis and treatment | BMJ Best Practice. [online] Available at: https://bestpractice.bmj.com/topics/en-gb/3000083.
2. McKnight, C.L. and Bracken Burns (2019). Pneumothorax. [online] Nih.gov. Available at: https://www.ncbi.nlm.nih.gov/books/NBK441885/.